Overcoming Childhood Obesity

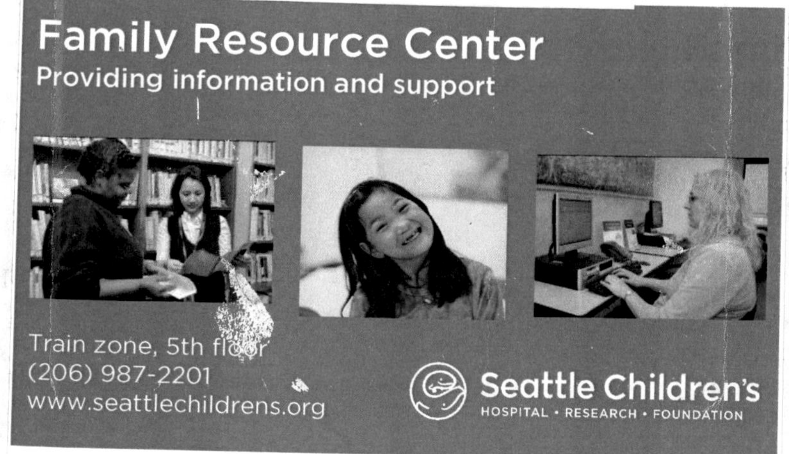

Bull Publishing Company
P.O. Box 1377
Boulder, CO 80304
800-676-2855
www.bullpub.com

ISBN 0-923521-78-X

Manufactured in the United States of America

Library of Congress Cataloging-in-Publication Data

Thompson, Colleen A.
Overcoming childhood obesity / by Colleen Thompson and Ellen Shanley.
p. cm.
Includes bibliographical references and index.
ISBN 0-923521-78-X
1. Obesity in children. 2. Obesity in children—Prevention. 3. Children—Nutrition. I. Shanley, Ellen L. II. Title.

RJ399.C6T48 2004
618.92'398—dc22

2003020379

Overcoming Childhood Obesity

Colleen A. Thompson, MS, RD

Ellen L. Shanley, MBA, RD, CD-N

University of Connecticut

College of Agriculture & Natural Resources

Department of Nutritional Sciences

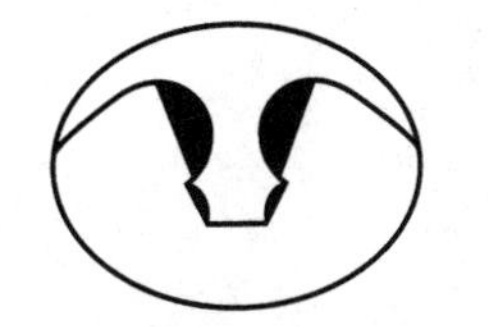

Bull Publishing Company

Boulder, Colorado

Dedication

For the love, support, continual patience,

and encouragement of our families:

Brian, Alexander, Kevin, and Eric Thompson

Peter, Amanda, and Gregg Shanley

CONTENTS

PREFACE

Thank you for taking time out of your busy lives to read this book! You are obviously committed to your child's health and well-being. We hope that reading and enjoying this book will be your first step on the road to a healthy active lifestyle for you and your family.

We'd like to make some suggestions to help you get the most out of the book. While you may be tempted to jump to the chapter focusing on the age of your own child/children, we think it would be most helpful for you to start with Chapter 1. In this first chapter, you'll learn what "obesity" really is, especially as it relates to children. You'll also read about the increased incidence of obesity in adults and kids in the United States. And you'll find out more about the physical and emotional consequences of being overweight for children. Finally, the vital role of parents and family in the prevention and treatment of obesity will be discussed. You, the parent, hold the key to improving the health and well-being of your children and your family as a whole.

Following Chapter 1 is a brief chapter about the basics of nutrition. This chapter answers the question, "What is healthy eating?" in a user-friendly format. Once you're armed with some of these basic facts, you'll be ready to go to the chapter or chapters that address the specific needs of children in various age groups. As you probably know, feeding a picky toddler is far different from dealing with the hectic schedule of an independent teenager. In Chapters 3, 4, and 5, you'll find practical advice that relates to the unique concerns of children of all ages—from babies to teens.

Chapter 6 follows the age group chapters. Its unique "Frequently Asked Questions" (FAQ's) format allows us to directly address some of the most common concerns parents have. In this chapter you'll learn about vegetarianism, eating disorders, and healthy snacking along with other important topics. After learning the basics you'll be ready to start planning healthy family meals. We've developed some simple menus and recipes with busy parents like you in mind. In Chapters 7 and 8, you'll find quick menu items, shortcuts, and tips for increasing the nutritional value of meals, and suggestions and hints for success. We've even provided shopping lists, suggestions for kitchen staples to have on hand, and easy-to-make recipes complete with nutrient analysis.

The final section of the book features resources and useful appendixes. While this is the last section of the book, it is certainly an important and useful one. This section is full of excellent and appropriate resources to help you find out more about topics related to childhood obesity. The appendixes contain useful charts and current dietary recommendations to help you assess your child's risk of overweight. Everyone needs a little guidance when making positive changes in their families' lives.

We would like to take this opportunity to thank a few people who helped us with recipe development and testing. Our special thanks go out to the following University of Connecticut Nutritional Sciences students: Marissa Ciorciari, Candice Jones, and Nicole Moretti. Finally, we would like to thank the dedicated staff at Bull Publishing, especially Jim Bull and our wonderful editor, Erin Mulligan.

Enjoy the book!
Colleen & Ellen

CHAPTER 1

Starting at the Beginning: With Parents

What's All the Fuss about Childhood Obesity?

During the past 20 years there has been a dramatic increase in obesity in the United States. Among adults, **obesity** has nearly **doubled,** increasing from approximately 15 percent in 1980 to an estimated 27 percent in 1999.[1]

Alarming as the data on American adults is, the picture is even bleaker when we look at the data on children. Obesity rates among children have skyrocketed. Let's look at some startling statistics.

- At least one child in five is overweight.
- The percentage of children who are overweight has more than doubled since 1970.
- The percentage of African American and Hispanic children who are overweight has increased by 120% since 1986.
- Almost 8% of four- and five-year-old children are overweight, nearly twice as many as 20 years ago.
- Childhood obesity is recognized as a national epidemic.[2]

The Health Costs

With this increase in overweight among children, we are beginning to see a corresponding increased incidence of adult diseases in these kids. For example, Type 2 diabetes, once considered to be an adult-onset disease, is now being diagnosed in children. As many as 30,000 children have Type 2 diabetes. Twenty-seven percent of children, who are not considered overweight, have one or more adverse cardiovascular disease risk factors. Of children who are considered overweight, nearly 61% of them have more than one adverse cardiovascular disease risk factors, such as high blood pressure or high cholesterol.

In 2001, The Surgeon General of the United States called for immediate action to prevent and decrease overweight and obesity in children and adolescents.[3] Hospital costs for diseases related to childhood obesity have increased threefold in the past 20 years, according to a recent news brief published by the American Academy of Pediatrics.[4] Annual hospital costs associated with obesity have increased from $35 million in 1979 to $127 million in 1999. The study also found that hospital visits for diseases related to obesity increased dramatically—diabetes nearly doubled, gallbladder disease tripled, and sleep apnea increased five-fold. The study's authors conclude that there is **a need for immediate diet and physical activity interventions to prevent continued weight gain in children.**

In addition to being a problem unto itself, childhood obesity is the first step in the progression into an overweight society. Overweight adolescents have a 70% chance of becoming overweight or obese adults. The likelihood is even greater if one or both parents is overweight or obese. Obese or overweight adults, like obese children, are at risk for a number of health problems including heart disease, diabetes, high blood pressure and certain cancers.

But the costs of being overweight for children and adolescents are not merely physical. The more immediate concern for young people is the social discrimination associated with obesity. Overweight kids generally have poor self-esteem and can suffer from depression.

The Emotional Costs

The emotional distress and low self-esteem of children suffering from chronic obesity is well-documented. Overweight children are often perceived as weak or lacking in self-control. A recent study in the *Journal of the American Medical Association* found that overweight kids report a poor quality of life. In fact, overweight children report a quality of life similar to that reported by young cancer patients on chemotherapy! These kids miss school more often due to weight-related ailments as well as having to endure teasing by their classmates. They are teased about their size and have trouble playing sports.[5]

For adolescents, being overweight during a time of life when most people are intensely preoccuped with appearance can lead to poor self-image. These teens become socially isolated, may suffer from delayed psychosocial development, and have trouble relating to their peers. Compared with women who were of normal weight in their teens, women who were overweight as teens had higher poverty rates, lower household income, fewer completed years of school, and were less likely to be married.[6]

Emotional costs such as these clearly demonstrate a need for intervention. Ideally, childhood obesity should be prevented using the strategies in this book with an emphasis on family-centered improvements in nutrition and physical activity habits. When overweight is already a problem in the household, it must be aggressively and sensitively treated with professional guidance.

What Exactly Is Obesity?

Obesity, especially childhood obesity, is a sensitive subject. Obesity for children is not defined in the same way as it is for adults. That's because adults are essentially "static." That is, adults have reached their adult height and should be striving to maintain a healthy weight for that height. Children, on the other hand, are still growing. Looking at their weight for height is not always useful at a single point in time. Their height continues to change over time. In fact, many health professionals prefer not to use the term "obese" in relation to children at all. According to the Centers for Disease Control (CDC), "Due to potential negative connotations associated with the term 'obesity', 'overweight' is preferred."[7]

To begin the discussion, we'll define the term "obesity" for adults. Then, we'll talk about the special concerns related to growing children.

Obesity in Adults

The most widely accepted tool used by health professionals to screen for obesity is the Body Mass Index (BMI). The BMI relates an adult's weight to their height using the equation (weight in kg)/(height in m)^2. Don't worry if your math is a little rusty! Most BMI graphs have done the math for you. Look at Figure 1.1 to find your BMI. Once you've figured out your BMI, you can see which category of "health risk" is associated with that number. The categories are as follows:

- Underweight: BMI < 18
- Healthy weight: BMI 19–24.9
- Overweight: BMI 25–29.9
- Obese: BMI >30

According to the National Institutes of Health, adults over age 18 who have a BMI greater than 25 are at risk

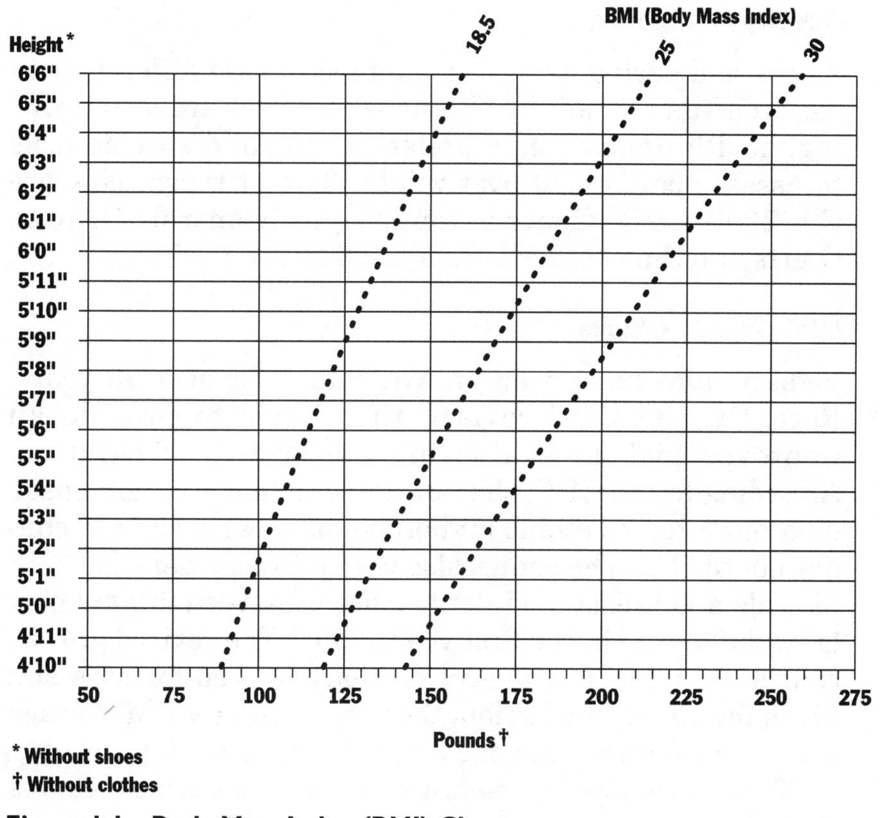

Figure 1.1 Body Mass Index (BMI) Chart

for premature death and disabilities as a result of being overweight or obese. We use the BMI because it is more highly correlated with body fat than other indicators of height and weight. Nevertheless, BMI is just a screening tool. It does not actually measure body fat. Body fat requires a much more sophisticated test done by trained professionals. It is possible to have a BMI in the "overweight" range, but not be considered at risk for chronic health conditions. This would be the case for a fit athlete whose body fat is low but whose weight, due to significant amount of muscle, may be in the "overweight" range for his or her height.

Obesity in Children

As we said earlier, obesity is defined a little differently in children than in adults. Because children are still growing, health professionals prefer to use child-specific tools to assess obesity and overweight. Two of these tools are the 2000 CDC (Centers for Disease Control) Growth charts and the new BMI-for-age charts.

CDC Growth Charts

Pediatricians have used growth charts for over 25 years. Recently, the CDC revised the charts to provide an improved tool for evaluating the growth of children. According to the CDC, the new growth charts "...are based on a more recent ethnic and economic cross-section of children in the US. The charts also take into consideration both formula and breast-fed infants since breast-fed infants may grow differently in the first year of life." The revised growth charts consist of 14 age-specific charts (seven for boys and seven for girls). In addition, there are two new BMI-for-age charts, one for boys and one for girls, ages 2 to 20 years old.

The charts are in essence a series of percentile curves that show the distribution of certain body measurements (i.e., height, weight, and head circumference) in American children. A child's growth can be tracked over time using these charts. Your pediatrician or other health care professional is best trained to do this. They can look for changes in these percentiles that may be cause for concern. For example, a child who is consistently at the 25th percentile for weight-for-age and suddenly jumps to the 75th percentile without a big jump in height might be at risk for being overweight. The health care provider should also monitor for significant drops in percentiles, which may mean that a child is not growing adequately. A pediatrician hopes to see a continual steady growth for a child and also hopes to see a child in similar percentiles for both height and weight. For example, a child who is in the 75th percentile for height-for-age should be close to the 75th percentile for weight-for-age.

An example of one of the growth charts showing a healthy pattern of growth is shown in Figure 1.2. Please keep in mind that there are many healthy patterns of

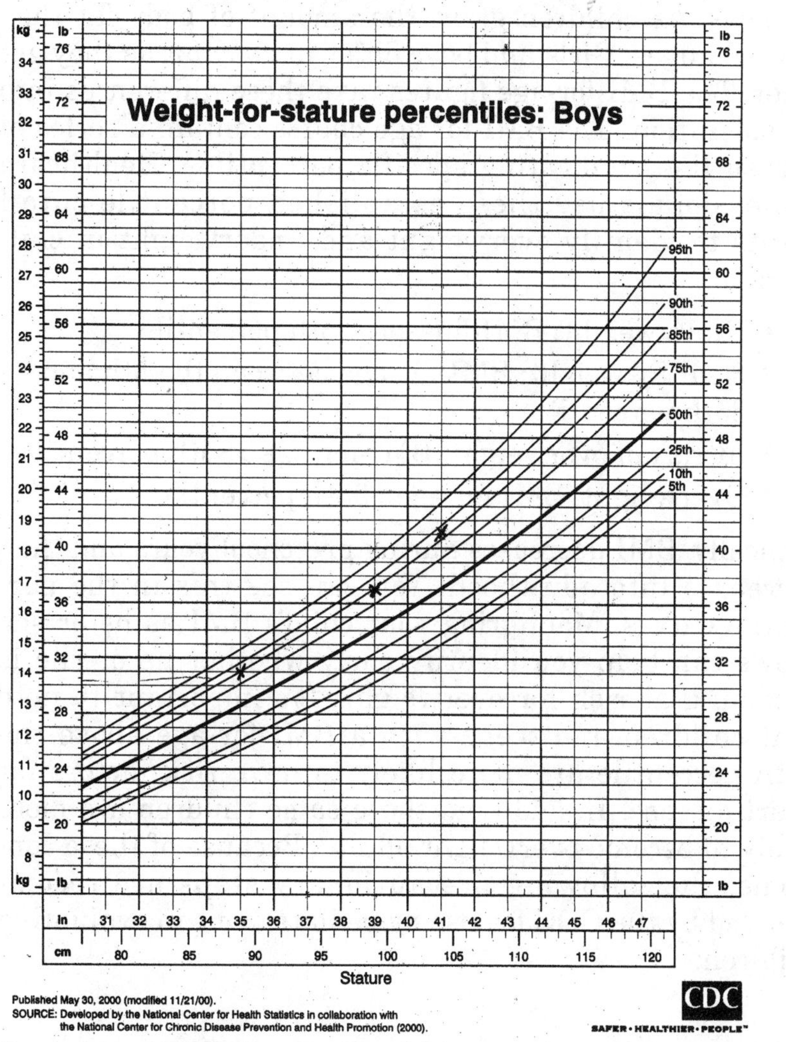

Figure 1.2 A CDC Growth Chart Showing a Healthy Pattern of Growth

growth. This is just one example. We've included blank growth charts in Appendix 1 for your convenience. If you monitor your child's growth using these charts, it is always a good idea to share any concerns you may have with your health care provider.

BMI–for–Age Charts

There are two BMI-for-age charts, one for girls and one for boys. As children grow, the amount of body fat they have changes. Girls and boys differ in body fat as they get older. The BMI-for-age figures take these differences into consideration. The BMI-for-age charts contain a series of curved lines indicating specific percentiles. Healthcare professionals use these established percentile cutoff points to identify overweight and underweight in children: [8]

- Underweight: BMI-for-age < 5th percentile
- Healthy weight: BMI-for-age between the 5th and 85th percentile
- At risk of overweight: BMI-for-age >85th percentile
- Overweight: BMI for age >95th percentile

Typically, BMI decreases during preschool years and then increases into adulthood. You can see this in the percentile curves. Monitoring your child's BMI as he or she grows can help you identify early whether he or she is becoming at risk for overweight. It's important to note that children and teens with a BMI-for-age above the 95th percentile are more likely to have risk factors for heart disease. In addition, those same children are more likely to become overweight adults. Because of these concerns, the following precautionary steps are recommended by the CDC for use by pediatricians in evaluating children:

- Children older than two with BMIs at or above the 95th percentile for age and sex are considered overweight, and should receive an in-depth assessment by the health care professional.
- Children older than two with BMIs between the 85th and 95th percentiles for age and sex are considered at-risk, and should be evaluated looking for any accompanying risk factors such as high blood pressure, high cholesterol, or diabetes.
- Children with an annual increase of two or more BMI units should be further evaluated by the health care professional.

Figures 1.3 and 1.4 show examples of completed BMI-for-age charts. Figure 1.3 shows the numbers for a healthy growing boy. You can see his BMI-for-age is within the range considered healthy and stays relatively constant over time. Figure 1.4 shows a female who is starting to show signs of overweight. Her BMI-for-age is within the healthy range at an early age but begins to rise as she gets older.

Knowing your child's BMI can be useful. However, you must remember to work with your health care professional. They are better qualified to diagnose your child as overweight or at risk for overweight. A blank BMI-for-age chart is in Appendix 2. Don't forget to look at BMI as children age, not at just a single point in their lives!

Why Is this Increase in Obesity Happening?

There is no single factor that ultimately is responsible for this increase in obesity in American children and adults. Rather, it is a unique combination of factors, each of which must be addressed in order for us to be successful at reducing and preventing obesity. Recognizing some of the key factors contributing to the problem is a good start. For the most part, obesity is caused by unhealthy eating behaviors and a sedentary lifestyle.

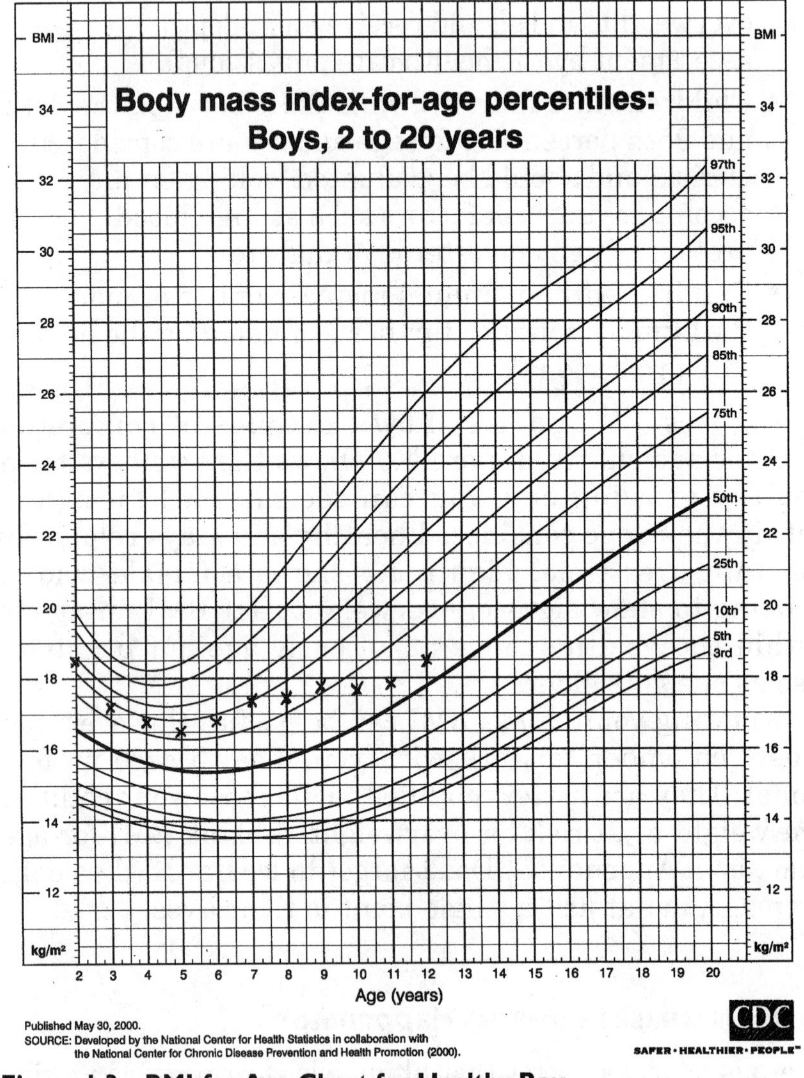
CDC Growth Charts: United States
Body mass index-for-age percentiles:
Boys, 2 to 20 years
BMI
34
32
30
28
26
24
22
20
18
16
14
12
kg/m²
97th
95th
90th
85th
75th
50th
25th
10th
5th
3rd
2
3
4
5
6
7
8
9
10
11
12
13
14
15
16
17
18
19
20
Age (years)
Published May 30, 2000.
SOURCE: Developed by the National Center for Health Statistics in collaboration with
the National Center for Chronic Disease Prevention and Health Promotion (2000).
CDC
SAFER • HEALTHIER • PEOPLE™

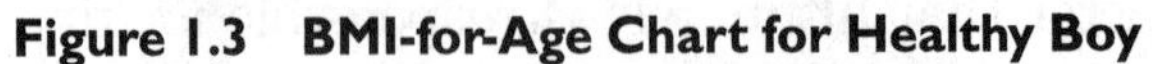

Figure 1.3 BMI-for-Age Chart for Healthy Boy

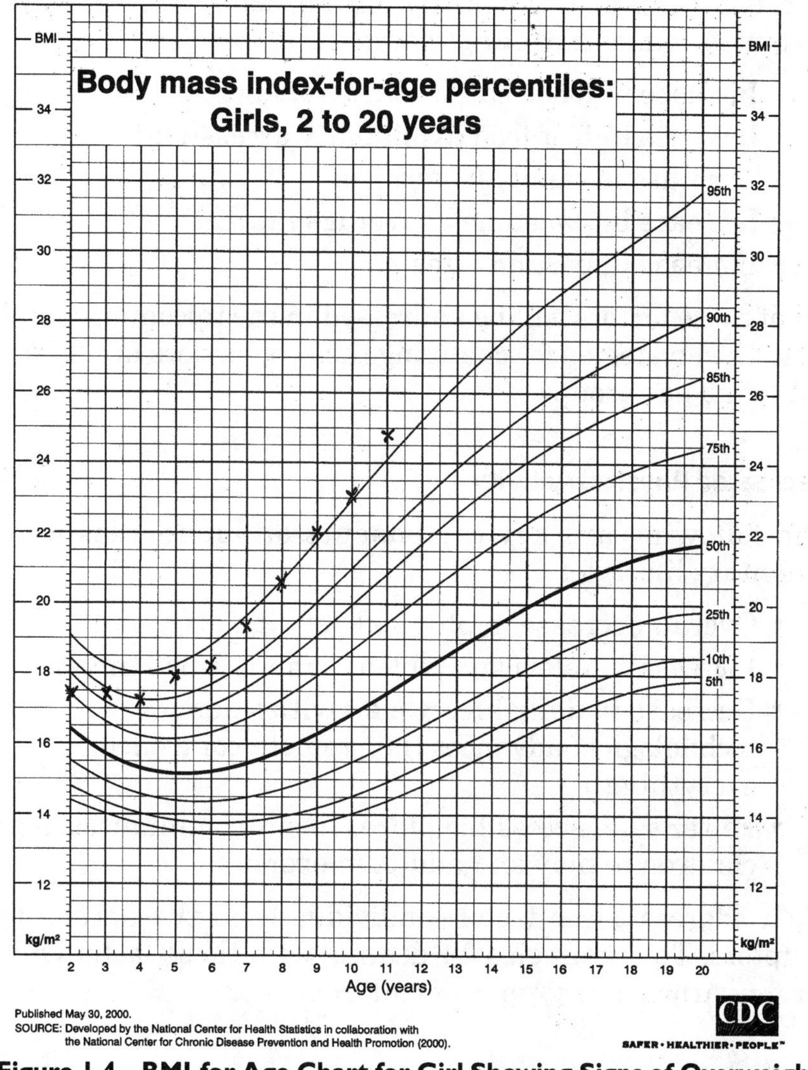

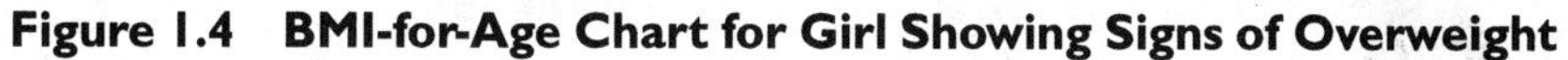

Figure 1.4 BMI-for-Age Chart for Girl Showing Signs of Overweight

Unhealthy Eating Behaviors

The following are unhealthy eating behaviors that are becoming common in our society:

- Increase in foods eaten away from home
- Increase in fast food availability/accessibility
- Decrease in family mealtimes
- Increase in sweetened beverage intake
- Increase in portion sizes

All of these factors will be addressed in the upcoming chapters. The strategies for changing these behaviors are different for all age groups.

Decreased Physical Activity

The following are key components of our increasingly sedentary lifestyle:

- Overall decrease in physical activity
- Increase in television, video, computer-use time
- Decrease in daily lifestyle activities due to technological advances (i.e., remote-controlled everything!)
- Fewer safe, accessible places in our communities for children to play and adults to exercise

We'll address these factors individually in the upcoming chapters. The strategies for dealing with these factors differ for various age groups of children.

Genetics

You may ask, "Doesn't genetics have anything to do with it?" (or "I'm overweight, won't my kids be overweight, too?") Individuals with a family history of obesity are two to three times more likely to be obese. We certainly can inherit our body type. Take a look at your parents and you may very well see your own body type. Children whose parents are overweight are more likely to become overweight themselves. However, someone who is genetically predisposed to obesity (i.e., obesity runs in their families) may never become obese if they choose a healthy diet and engage in regular physical activity. At the same time, someone who is not genetically predisposed to obesity (i.e., obesity does not run in their families) may become obese if they eat a diet too high in calories and get little exercise.

Genetics alone cannot explain the sudden increase in obesity. Environmental factors such as the dramatic increased availability of high-calorie foods combined with a drastic drop in regular physical activity do seem to offer more of an explanation. Obese families tend to consume more calories and exercise less than lean families. You and your children may not have control over an inherited body type, but you do have control over how healthy that body can be. You may not be destined to wear a size four, but maintaining a healthy weight for your height and age is certainly possible regardless of what genes you have inherited.

What Can We Do?

There is no "cure" for obesity. In fact, obesity can be a life-long problem. No magic pills or potions exist! Dieting is a multi-billion dollar industry with consumers trying anything and everything to lose weight. Unfortunately, the majority of dieters are not successful at losing the weight and keeping it off. With children, ***dieting is not recommended.*** Reducing calories in a child's diet can compromise their growth and overall health. However, positive changes in eating behaviors and physical activity can improve a child's health and decrease his or her risk of becoming overweight or obese as an adult.

Since the causes of obesity are so varied, so must be the solutions. The best "cure" is prevention. A good place to begin implementing a prevention plan is at home. This book will focus on the prevention of obesity at various stages of the lifecycle from infancy through the teenage years. Strategies for improving the nutritional status of kids will be provided, with an emphasis on increasing physical activity and on the importance of the family unit.

The Importance of the Family

It is the family piece that can have the most impact on obesity prevention. From family walks to family bike rides to family food shopping and family meal preparation, getting kids and their families up and moving and working together to choose and prepare healthy meals can be the beginning of life-long healthy changes. Making the commitment to positive change as a family can make a huge difference in the health and well-being of our children. Something as simple (and enjoyable) as eating together as a family more often can directly and positively affect what and how much kids eat. See Table 1.1 for more interesting facts about how we eat and what we eat.

This book will not offer a "diet" for a child to "go on." Rather, we recommend family-centered changes in eating behaviors and lifestyle that will have a lasting impact, resulting in healthier, more active kids and families. These healthier, active kids will lose excess weight as they continue to grow and develop into healthy, active adults. Such changes cannot be possible without the *whole* family adopting these behaviors. This means that the parents must be role models for the children. Healthy eating and daily physical activity are learned behaviors. Parents are the best teachers!

It's important that any changes made be made in a positive manner. Given what we know about poor self-esteem in overweight children, it's vital to encourage healthy behaviors in a positive and nurturing way. The goal is to make children feel good about themselves in the process. It's also important that any changes be made for the whole family, not just the overweight child. The child mustn't feel singled out or isolated. After all, healthy eating and regular physical activity are good for everyone!

Table 1.1 Eating Habits in Today's Families

Higher frequency of television viewing during dinner is associated with a lower fruit and vegetable consumption and higher fat consumption.
At least one in three families report that they are too busy to eat dinner together.
Arguments during dinner are associated with higher fat consumption.
Foods eaten at home tend to be lower in fat and higher in fiber, calcium and iron than foods eaten away from home.
Consumption of food prepared away from home increased from 18% of total calories in 1978 to 32% of total calories in 1996.
Women who are reluctant to try new foods are more likely to have daughters with similar aversions.
Finicky eaters eat fewer vegetables daily.
Sweetened beverages make up 51% of kids' daily liquid intake.
Sixty-five % of kids who "surf the Web" daily eat while online.
More overweight kids report eating dinner while watching TV than their normal-weight peers.

Sources:

1. Centers for Disease Control. *Obesity trends: Obesity trends among adults — 1985–2001.* Retrieved August 26, 2003 from http://www.cdc.gov/nccdphp/dnpa/obesity/trend/index.htm.
2. Ogden, C., Flegal, K., Carroll, M., & Johnson, C. (2000). Prevalence and trends in overweight among US children and adolescents. *Journal of the American Medical Association,* 288, 1728–1732.
3. Superintendent of Documents. *The Surgeon General's call to action to prevent and decrease overweight and obesity–recommendations for schools* (Item number 017-001-00551-7) Washington, DC: U.S. Government Printing Office.
4. Guijing, W. & Dietz, W.H. (2002). Economic burden of obesity in youths aged 6 to 17 years: 1979–1999. *Pediatrics,* 109, e81.
5. Schwimmer, J.B., Burwinkle, T.M., & Varni, J.W. (2003). Health-related quality of life of severely obese children and adolescents. *Journal of the American Medical Association,* 289, 1813–1819.

6. Gortmaker, S.L., Must, A., Perrin, J.M., Sobol, A.M., & Dietz, W.H. (1993). Social and economic consequences of overweight in adolescence and young adulthood. *New England Journal of Medicine,* 329,1008–1012.
7. Centers for Disease Control. (May 2000). CDC growth chart training. Retrieved August 26, 2003 from http://www.cdc.gov/nccdphp/dnpa/growthcharts/training/modules/module3/text/page1b.htm.
8. Centers for Disease Control. (2000). Body Mass Index-for-Age (children): BMI is used differently with children than it is with adults. Retrieved August 26, 2003 from http://www.cdc.gov/nccdphp/dnpa/bmi/bmi-for-age.htm.

CHAPTER 2

Getting Started with the Basics

What Is Healthy Eating?

In Chapter 1, you read the alarming statistics and learned about the emotional and physical consequences of children and adults being overweight. You learned how to assess overweight using the appropriate tools. Regardless of what BMI you or your children have, learning to balance healthy eating with regular physical activity is beneficial for all of us!

A healthy diet is based on whole grains, fruits, vegetables, milk, and meat or meat substitutes. It is a diet that includes a wide variety of foods that we all can enjoy. Unfortunately, choosing those foods has become increasingly difficult in recent years. There are so many choices and so much information on what to eat and what not to eat that it is easy to become confused.

It's time to get back to a few basics. Just as there are recommendations for a healthy weight, there are recommendations for a healthy diet. There are two common tools most often used to assess the adequacy of the

American diet, the Dietary Guidelines for Americans and the Food Guide Pyramid.

The Dietary Guidelines

Every five years or so, the United States Department of Agriculture and the Department of Health and Human Services issue the Dietary Guidelines for Americans.

The guidelines are just that—guidelines. The mission of the Dietary Guidelines 2000 is "to provide positive, simple and consistent messages to help consumers achieve healthy, active lifestyles." The guidelines are general in nature, allowing the consumer choice and flexibility when it comes to their diet.

The guidelines are a set of nutrition recommendations designed to promote healthy eating for Americans and to prevent or reduce nutrition-related diseases. For example, research has shown that a diet high in fiber is associated with a decreased risk of certain cancers and other chronic diseases. Therefore, the Dietary Guidelines recommend a diet that includes plenty of whole grains, fruits, and vegetables, all of which are good sources of fiber.

The *Dietary Guidelines for Americans 2000* carry three basic messages—the ABC's for your health—as illustrated in Figure 2.1.

A. Aim for fitness

B. Build a healthy base

C. Choose Sensibly

By following the guidelines that accompany these basic messages, you and your family can enjoy a healthy diet and lifestyle; making choices that work for you while you all enjoy eating.

Let's look at each message and its accompanying guideline. In this book, we suggest some strategies to help you follow these guidelines and incorporate them into

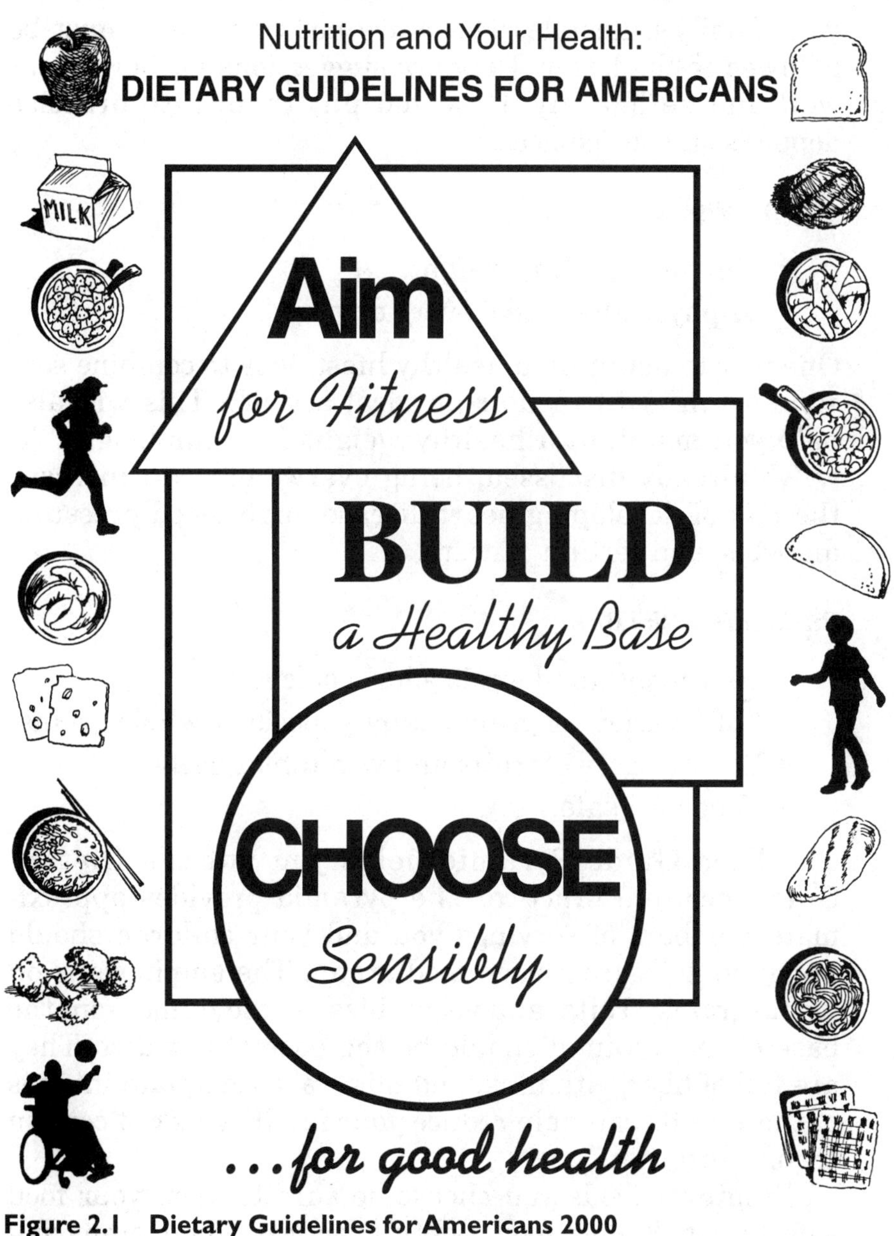

Figure 2.1 Dietary Guidelines for Americans 2000

your family's lifestyle. These are not rules that must be followed to the letter. They are suggestions for how to eat well and be healthy. How you put them into practice depends on your choices.

Aim for Fitness

- Aim for a healthy weight.
- Be physically active every day.

One way to maintain a healthy lifestyle is to combine sensible eating with regular physical activity. This will also help you maintain a healthy weight for your height. As we've already discussed, being overweight can increase the risk of developing heart disease, high blood pressure, diabetes, and certain cancers.

Build a Healthy Base

- Let the pyramid guide your food choices.
- Eat a variety of grains daily, especially whole grains.
- Eat a variety of fruits and vegetables daily.
- Keep food safe.

The Food Guide Pyramid helps you put the Dietary Guidelines into practice. The pyramid provides approximate numbers of servings you and your children should consume daily from each food group. The emphasis is on whole grains, fruits, and vegetables. These items from the base of the pyramid should be the base of our diet. They are full of fiber, vitamins, and minerals. Adequate intakes of these foods can help reduce your family's risk of certain chronic diseases.

Whatever foods you choose be sure to keep your food safe to eat. Follow food safety practices when preparing and storing food. You can protect your family from food-borne illness and contamination.

Choose Sensibly

- Choose a diet that is low in saturated fat and cholesterol and moderate in total fat.
- Choose beverages and foods that allow you to limit your intake of sugars.
- Choose and prepare foods with less salt.
- If you drink alcoholic beverages, do so in moderation.

Eating is all about making choices. If you and your family choose sensibly, you greatly increase your chances of leading healthy, productive, and active lives. Choosing moderate size portions of foods lower in fat, saturated fat, and cholesterol may help reduce your risk of developing heart disease. Limiting your intake of sugars will reduce your risk of tooth decay and also increase the likelihood that you will choose more nutritious foods. Sugar often takes the place of more nutritious foods in our diet. For example, soda is made almost entirely from sugar and has very few nutrients. Having a glass of low-fat milk instead of soda will provide similar amounts of calories but will give your children calcium, protein, and other nutrients as well.

Members of your family may also need to limit the salt in their diet, particularly if they have a tendency towards high blood pressure. If you don't know your blood pressure, you should have it checked. High blood pressure has no symptoms, but is very dangerous.

Finally, alcohol should not be consumed at all by young people.

The Food Guide Pyramid

The Food Guide Pyramid was developed to help people put the Dietary Guidelines into practice. While the

Dietary Guidelines give you general information about *how* to eat, the Food Guide Pyramid gives more specific guidance on *what* and *how much* to eat (see Figure 2.2).

The pyramid shape is significant in that it is designed to illustrate how each food group contributes to the diet. The base, or the largest part of the pyramid, contains the foods that are the foundation of our diet, that is, breads, cereals, rice, and pasta. We need about 6–11 servings each day from this group. A serving of pasta or rice is about the size of a computer mouse. The next level

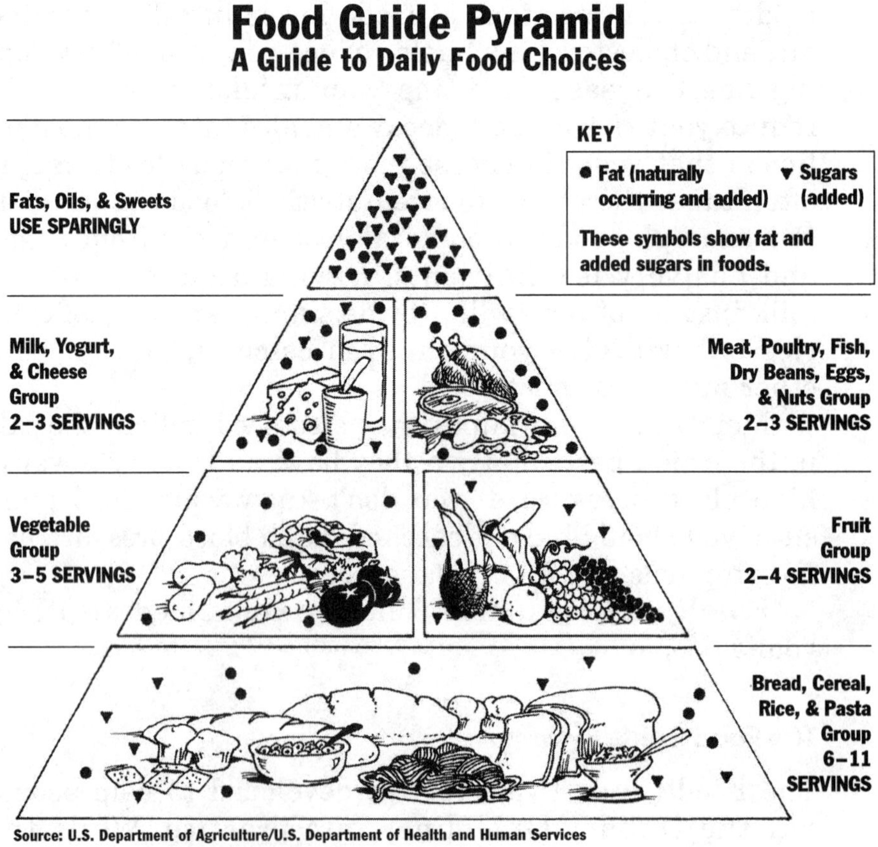

Food Guide Pyramid
A Guide to Daily Food Choices

KEY
● Fat (naturally occurring and added) ▼ Sugars (added)
These symbols show fat and added sugars in foods.

Fats, Oils, & Sweets
USE SPARINGLY

Milk, Yogurt, & Cheese Group
2–3 SERVINGS

Meat, Poultry, Fish, Dry Beans, Eggs, & Nuts Group
2–3 SERVINGS

Vegetable Group
3–5 SERVINGS

Fruit Group
2–4 SERVINGS

Bread, Cereal, Rice, & Pasta Group
6–11 SERVINGS

Source: U.S. Department of Agriculture/U.S. Department of Health and Human Services

Figure 2.2 The Food Guide Pyramid

includes vegetables (3–5 servings/day) and fruits (2–4 servings/day). As the pyramid continues to decrease in size, the next level recommends 2–3 servings/day from the milk, yogurt, and cheese group and 2–3 servings per day from the meat, poultry, dry beans, eggs, and nuts group. A serving of meat is about the size of a deck of playing cards. There are no recommended servings for the small tip of the pyramid, which includes fats, oils and sweets. Our complete nutrient needs can be met with the rest of the pyramid, so the tip is for the extras. We should try to consume limited amounts of these items. Table 2.1 shows how you can fit in all of the foods in the pyramid and obtain the nutritional benefits associated with the foods from each group.

Table 2.1 Using the Food Guide Pyramid

Food Group/Serving Size	The Benefits	Examples
Breads, Cereals, Pasta and Rice, (6–11 servings/day) 1 slice bread 1/2 cup cooked cereal (like oatmeal) 1 ounce dry cereal 1/2 cup cooked pasta Choose whole grain whenever possible	The foods in this group provide plenty of tummy-filling fiber, energy-producing B vitamins, iron for red blood cells, and zinc to ward off sickness.	Whole grain cereal for breakfast (2 ounces = 2 servings) 2 slices of whole grain bread at lunch (2 servings) 1 bagel for a snack (1 bagel = 2 servings) 1 cup pasta with dinner (2 servings) Daily total = 8 servings
Vegetables (3–5 servings/day) 1/2 cup cooked or raw chopped vegetables 1 cup leafy vegetables 3/4 cup vegetable juice 10 French fries	Vegetables provide essential vitamins and disease-fighting antioxidants such as Vitamins A, C, and folate. They also provide fiber, minerals, and phytochemicals such as lycopene.	1/2 cup carrot sticks with lunch (1 serving) 1/2 cup lettuce and tomato on a sandwich (1 serving) 1 cup of cooked vegetables at dinner (2 servings) Daily total = 4 servings
Fruits (2–4 servings/day) 1 medium apple, banana, or orange 1/2 cup chopped, cooked or canned fruit 1 cup berries 3/4 cup fruit juice 1/4 cup dried fruit	Fruits provide vitamins A and C as well as good sources of filling fiber, potassium, and disease-fighting antioxidants.	3/4 cup 100% fruit juice at breakfast (1 serving) 1/2 banana or other fresh fruit on your cereal (1/2 serving) 1 apple with lunch (1 serving) 1/4 cup raisins for a snack (1 serving) Daily total = 3 1/2 servings

Table 2.1 Using the Food Guide Pyramid *(Continued)*

Food Group/Serving Size	The Benefits	Examples
Milk, Yogurt, and Cheese (2–3 servings/day) 1 cup milk or yogurt 1 1/2 ounces natural cheese 2 ounces processed cheese 1 1/2 cups ice cream 1 cup frozen yogurt 2 cups cottage cheese	This group provides calcium, vitamin D, protein and riboflavin, all important in bone health	1/2 cup milk with cereal (1/2 serving) 1 cup yogurt for snack or treat yourself to 1 cup of ice cream (1 serving) 1 1/2 ounces of cheese with crackers for a snack (1 serving) Daily total = 2 1/2 servings
Meat, poultry, fish, dry beans, eggs, and nuts (2–3 servings/day) 2–3 ounces cooked lean meat, poultry or fish 2–3 eggs 4–6 tablespoons peanut butter 1 1/2 cups cooked dry beans 1 cup nuts	This group offers plenty of high quality protein as well as iron, B vitamins, and zinc. All of these are important for strengthening immunity and building strong muscles.	2 ounces lean deli meat on a sandwich (1 serving) 3 ounces lean meat at dinner (1 serving) 1/2 cup nuts for a snack (1/2 serving) Daily total = 2 1/2 servings
Fats, oils and sweets (use sparingly) butter, mayonnaise, salad dressing, jelly, jam, candies	Just extra calories, few nutrients.	Choose these items as extras and not as the base for your diet.

Since the introduction of the traditional Food Guide Pyramid, many other pyramids have been developed to reflect the diverse needs and make-up of our society. For example, there is a vegetarian pyramid. There are several pyramids reflecting various ethnicities such as the African American Pyramid, the Latino American Pyramid, and the Asian American Pyramid. These pyramids use the same shape and have a similar nutritional emphasis as the traditional pyramid, but include foods that are commonly consumed by the appropriate populations. There is even an activity pyramid and a pyramid for young children.

The traditional pyramid has recently been criticized by some for not reflecting newer scientific knowledge about healthy fats and oils (such as fish oils, certain plant oils, etc.), whole grains, and legumes. In addition, some of the newer thinking suggests including water and daily exercise in the base of the pyramid. Part of the problem with the Food Guide Pyramid is the inconsistent application of the recommended serving sizes.

We've included examples in Appendix 3 of some of these other pyramids. What's important in all the pyramids is the emphasis on overall healthy eating and the inclusion of a wide variety of foods. Of course, no one can be perfect when it comes to eating. Fortunately you don't need to be. *All* foods can certainly fit into a healthy diet. It's really about choices and portions of foods. You needn't deprive yourself of any one food or food group. Rather, rethink your family's consumption of foods that don't have a lot of nutrient value like candy, chips, and soda and focus on increasing consumption of foods with lots of nutritional value like whole grains, fruits, and vegetables.

Dietary Reference Intakes (DRI's)

The Dietary Guidelines and the Food Guide Pyramid provide information on how to eat as well as what *foods* and how much of certain *foods* to eat. For those wanting to know the amounts of specific essential *nutrients* required by the body, the government recently established a set of reference values known as the Dietary Reference Intakes or DRI's. The DRI's are estimates of nutrient intakes to be used in planning and assessing healthy diets. The DRI's include both recommended intakes and limits for upper intakes. This information is provided to insure that people know how much of a particular nutrient is healthy to consume, thereby preventing excessive consumption.

Prior to the development of the DRI's, the Recommended Dietary Allowances (RDA's) were the standards used. However, the RDA's were formulated with the prevention of deficiencies in mind. Since true nutrient deficiencies are now rare in the US, the RDA's have become less useful to the general public. In addition, there is a greater recognition of the need to decrease the incidence of chronic diseases through better nutrition. The DRI's include levels for nutrients that may reduce the risk of heart disease, certain cancers and other diet-related diseases. Appendix 4 provides an overview of the DRI's for various nutrients.

Implementing Changes

Now you are armed with the facts on obesity and some information on recommendations for a healthy diet. You may even feel ready to make some changes in your family's eating habits. However, change is never easy, especially when it comes to children. Parents often meet with resistance when introducing new foods or suggesting that the television be turned off. As your child grows, the issues surrounding food and physical activity change. Recognizing this, we have identified key nutrition and physical activity issues for various age groups. The upcoming chapters will offer assistance in addressing these issues taking into consideration the diverse needs of each age group.

CHAPTER 3

Creating a Healthy Environment for Your Young Child

Infants, Toddlers, and Preschoolers

Anna is a healthy active preschooler who has suddenly decided she will only eat macaroni & cheese for lunch and dinner every day. Mom is starting to worry that her daughter isn't getting enough nutrition. Her mom is trying everything to get Anna to eat a more balanced diet. Mom is coaxing and bribing Anna to try other foods, but Anna is stubborn! The more frustrated and controlling Mom gets, the more willful and inflexible Anna becomes. What to do???

Your Young Child and Food

Children and food. What a unique, and wonderful (and sometimes frustrating) relationship! From the moment a child is born, food serves as both nourishment and comfort. Often, feeding a child seems to be the most natural part of parenting. We love to feed them when they are babies. If you have had the opportunity to breastfeed, it is likely that you found it to be a very meaningful encounter. Bottle-feeding a newborn is also very fulfilling as you hold your baby close and see your child comforted and happy.

We love to watch our children eat and see them grow. Sometimes, though, we develop concerns as children began to assert their independence and have a greater say in what goes in their little mouths.

It may seem that obesity shouldn't be a problem in toddlers and preschoolers, but the incidence is definitely rising. As we said in Chapter 1, almost 8% of four- and five-year-old children are overweight, nearly double that of 20 years ago.[1] The good news is that these preschool years are the times when changes are most easily made in a child's eating and exercise behavior. Young children are still eager to please their parents. They also tend to imitate the behaviors that they see. If the behaviors they are exposed to include healthy eating and regular physical activity, youngsters will be very likely to adopt them. Of course, the opposite is also true. Even young children notice if excessive television watching, snacking, and sedentary behaviors are the norm in a house. Bad habits are just as likely to rub off on them as good and they will quickly adapt to what they see.

As the chapter-opening story illustrates, feeding young children can be tricky. It can be particularly frustrating for a parent when children are picky about food or seem to be eating too much or not enough. As challenging as it may seem, making the effort to feed your child a healthy and nutritious diet is worth it. Developing good eating and physical activity habits when children are young sets the stage for healthier behaviors as they grow.

This chapter will identify key factors related to healthy eating and physical activity in infants, toddlers, and preschoolers. We will also discuss the special demands you face as parents of children in this age group. Our goal is to give you enough information to help you and your family successfully and happily negotiate the dinner (and lunch and breakfast and snack) table during the early childhood years.

Top Ten Healthy Behaviors

The following list features behaviors that we feel can make all the difference as you help your child make the daily decisions about food and activity that will lead to habit-forming good behaviors.

1. Infants are breast-fed if possible.
2. Children regularly eat with the family.
3. A variety of foods is offered at mealtimes.
4. Mealtimes are a pleasant part of the family routine.
5. Excess juice and sweetened beverages are limited.
6. Fast food is limited.
7. Children are encouraged to feed themselves at an appropriate age.
8. All family members including children exercise daily.
9. Television/computer/video game time is limited for all family members.
10. Parents serve as role models for healthy eating and regular physical activity.

Infants Are Breast-Fed If Possible

Exclusive breast-feeding (without the introduction of juice, solids, or formula) for the first six months is the ideal feeding pattern for infants. The benefits are many, for both the child and the mother. Children benefit from the special nutrition as well as the natural antibodies in breast milk that provide protection from illness. Benefits for moms include greater fat loss after pregnancy and reduced rates of pre-menopausal breast and ovarian cancers.

Breast-fed babies tend to be leaner than bottle-fed babies. Breast-fed babies also appear to have more control over how much they actually eat. This makes sense. Think about a breast-fed baby for a moment. Mom can't see how much milk the baby is actually getting. The baby stops sucking when he or she is full, and the mother usually accepts that decision. Studies have shown that with bottle-fed babies, moms tend to judge the baby's fullness by how much is left in the bottle. These babies are often encouraged to "finish" even when they may already be full. If allowed to choose when and how much to drink, infants are usually able to adjust their intake to meet their energy (caloric) needs. However, if the bottle is persistently put in the child's mouth, the child may end up consuming more calories than they need. This can also interfere with the baby's ability to recognize when he or she is truly full.

If you breast-feed your child, you have started them on a healthy path. Be sure to watch your baby for signs that he or she is full and pay attention to them. Don't force the baby to "finish" or keep sucking when they are showing signs of disinterest or fullness. If you are concerned about how much your baby is eating, talk to your health care professional. They should be tracking your child's growth on growth charts. With the aid of these charts, you can see how well your child is growing and you will become aware of any problems.

Special Concerns for the Bottle-fed Baby

If your child isn't being breast-fed, there are some things you can be doing to ensure a healthy well-fed baby.

Feed your baby a fortified infant formula. Pick one that you and your pediatrician agree is best for the baby.

Be sure to prepare the formula as directed. Don't add too much water. That will only make your baby hungrier and could lead to overhydration.

Bottle-feed on demand. Avoid regimented schedules. It is healthiest to let the baby decide when he or she is hungry.

Only feed your baby until he or she is full. If the infant is fussing and pushing the bottle away, he is done eating. Don't force him to finish the bottle.

Help your child find other ways to comfort him/herself when full. If a baby is fussy after meals, he may not be hungry; he may just need to suckle a little more. Help the baby find a thumb or offer a pacifier.

Children Regularly Eat with the Family

Families are more likely to eat a nutritious meal when most or all of the family eats together.[2] Children who eat with the family tend to make better food choices and learn to try new foods more readily than children who are fed separately. In addition to improved nutrition, studies show that other benefits of family mealtimes include better communication, stronger family bonds, and shared learning.

It's never too early to have a child begin to eat with the family. Once your baby has started on some solid food, try to include him or her at the table at every family meal. Their "dinner" could even be just a few Cheerios®! Pull the highchair up to the table. Offer them food if they are hungry. Even if they are not eating with the family or eating the same foods as the rest of the family yet, they are learning a lot by watching everyone enjoy their meal at the table and communicate with one another.

Once children have begun eating table foods, include them in the mealtime as often as possible. Offer them any appropriate foods that are being eaten by the rest of the family. Children imitate what they see. If they see you eat it, they will want to try it too! Simply make sure the food is safe for them to eat by mashing, pureeing, or cutting into small pieces to avoid any choking hazards.

It's important to take into consideration your children's physical and emotional development when it comes to mealtimes. Understanding their abilities will make it easier for you to plan meals accordingly and include them in the process. For example, recognizing when a child is ready to use a spoon or drink from a cup and offering the appropriate utensil can help foster feeding independence.

Janice Fletcher, Ed.D. and Laurel Branen, Ph.D., R.D. from the University of Idaho, College of Agriculture are nationally recognized experts on issues related to feeding children. In their work they have applied famed psychologist Erik Erikson's stages of development to feeding. Table 3.1 shows the developmental stages associated with early childhood and eating behaviors.

Table 3.1 Fletcher and Branen's Adaptation of Erikson's Psychosocial Stages Application for Children's Eating Skills Development

AGE: INFANT
STAGE: TRUST VERSUS MISTRUST Children develop feelings that they can rely on the consistency and security of the world around them.
FEEDING BEHAVIORS TRUST Adult sets a comfortable mood and tone, including securely holding and responding to the child, rather than propping bottles or group feeding children seated in high chairs. Adult provides appropriate foods when the baby shows hunger cues. Adult does not unnecessarily interrupt the child's focus on eating. Baby is fed when hungry. Adult stops feeding the baby when the baby shows that he/ she is through eating. Adult discerns which cues are hunger cues and which cues are indicators of other discomforts, refraining from using feeding as the answer to all cries. Adult stops feeding when baby turns away from the food. Adult determines that food temperature is appropriate.
MISTRUST (AVOID THESE STRATEGIES!) Adult feeds child on strict schedule, not in harmony with the child's hunger cues. Adult forces the nipple or spoon into a child's mouth. Adult feeds the child on every discomfort cue. In childcare settings, older babies are fed in a round robin fashion as they sit in high chairs. Adult moves from child to child on a rotation schedule determined by the adult, feeding each child mechanically.

Table 3.1 Fletcher and Branen's Adaptation of Erikson's Psychosocial Stages Application for Children's Eating Skills Development *(Continued)*

AGE: TODDLER

STAGE: AUTONOMY VERSUS SHAME AND DOUBT

Children have a sense that they exist as separate human beings. "I am! Look at ME," is the phrase to describe this stage.

FEEDING BEHAVIORS

AUTONOMY

Children are encouraged to feed themselves, regardless of mess.
Children may say no to foods.
Children may combine foods in the way they decide.
Children may go on food jags.
Child-sized portions of food are presented.
Food is served to children so that they can be successful, rather than frustrated. For example, pizza is cut into bite-sized pieces, rather than served as a slice.

SHAME AND DOUBT (AVOID THESE STRATEGIES!)

Adult feeds children even though the children have adequately developed grasps and finger control.
Adult takes over feeding when the children are eating messily.
Adult excessively interrupts the children's eating for hand and face-wiping.
Adult forces children to clean their plates and to eat all foods, with little regard to the children's hunger or satiety cues or individual preferences.
Adult serves child's plate with adult-sized portions.

AGE: EARLY CHILDHOOD

STAGE: INITIATIVE VERSUS GUILT

Child has a sense of taking risks as a safe behavior. "I will try" is the phrase that shows a healthy sense of initiative.

FEEDING BEHAVIORS

INITIATIVE

Adult accepts child's decision to stop eating when the child says, "I'm full."
Adult encourages child to determine how much, if any, of a new food to try.
Adult respects child's ability to dislike or like a new food.
Food is presented to the children so that they can serve themselves, deciding how much to put on their plates.
Spills are expected and treated as routine, rather than crisis.
Child sized utensils are provided so the child can more easily develop skills for feeding and serving self.

GUILT (AVOID THESE STRATEGIES!)

Child is chastised when he/she grows fatigued and sloppily uses utensils.
Adult scolds children for not cleaning their plates.
Child fails using utensils that are too big or heavy for his/her strength, balance, and endurance.
Child is scolded for spills.
Adult chastises or shows disappointment when a child shows dislike of foods.
Adult puts more on child's plate than the child can comfortably eat.

A Variety of Foods Is Offered at Mealtimes

It's wonderful to see children begin to assert their independence. Unfortunately, it is often at mealtime that children begin to do it! Getting children to try new foods, especially fruits and vegetables, can be extremely challenging for parents and caregivers. Young children have a natural fear of the unknown. It's not unusual, nor is it really a cause for concern, for a child to go on a "food jag" where they seem to want to eat only one or two foods. The children will usually grow out of it. However, the sooner you get kids to eat and enjoy a variety of foods, the greater the likelihood that they will learn to choose a more nutritious diet during the rest of their lives.

In the United States, fruit and vegetable intake among young children is abysmal. In fact, only 14% of kids eat the recommended servings per day of fruits and only 17% eat the recommended servings per day of vegetables. Since these foods offer plenty of nutrition for just a few calories, kids would benefit from increasing their intake of fruits and vegetables. So what to do if your little one turns up his nose?

Be patient. If you don't make too much of a fuss about it, kids will usually give up on food jags. The more of an issue you make, the more control the kids know they have.

Keep trying. Studies have shown that it takes 10–15 exposures to a new food before kids will accept it. Don't give up after the first try and assume the child just doesn't like it. Keep offering the food in small amounts. Kids taste with all of their senses, so it is quite normal for a young child to want to touch, smell and taste the food. They may even spit it out after tasting! This is OK. It is exposing them to the food and increasing the chance that they may accept it at some point.

Model positive behavior. Kids are more likely to try foods if they see someone else, especially a caregiver, eating the food. If you aren't eating fruits and vegetables, it is unlikely that your children will develop a taste for them.

Try different preparation methods. Kids' taste buds are far more sensitive than adults'. They may taste bitterness adults cannot in certain vegetables. Kids are also fussier when it comes to texture of foods. Some kids won't tolerate a cooked vegetable but will eat it raw. Experiment a little! Kids also love to eat with their hands. They will often eat something new if they can pick it up themselves.

Involve children in food preparation. Children are more likely to try something they have helped to prepare. They can help plant seeds in the garden or help pick the vegetables. Depending on their age, they can do various jobs in the kitchen such as mixing, chopping, or measuring.

Don't force children to eat. The caregiver can really only be responsible for providing nutritious food. You are not responsible for what and how much the child eats. Forcing them to eat serves to associate the food with negative pressure. Forcing children to eat also makes mealtime unpleasant. Food becomes less about nourishment and more about control. When this happens, kids start to associate food with unpleasantness and may end up with unhealthy eating behaviors.

Don't bribe, scold, or reward children with food. As stated earlier, when food becomes a control issue, eating becomes unhealthy and mealtimes become unpleasant. Rewarding children with food, i.e. giving dessert if they eat their vegetables, elevates dessert to a higher level. Children may then associate eating the vegetables with something difficult that must be done to get the reward. Some people tend to overeat later in life because as they were growing up they were not allowed dessert unless they finished the food on their plate!

Make sure portion sizes are appropriate for your child's age. Kids aren't mini-adults. Their portion sizes should be smaller and adults shouldn't expect them to eat the same amount of food as an adult. Table 3.2 lists suggested serving sizes for kids.

Table 3.2 Suggested Serving Sizes for Children

Breads & Grains	1–3 years old	4–6 years
bread	1/2 slice of bread	1 slice
cooked rice or pasta	1/4–1/3 cup	1/3–1/2 cup
cooked cereal	1/4–1/3 cup	1/3–1/2 cup
dry cereal	1/4–1/2 cup	1/2–3/4 cup
Vegetables		
Cooked or raw	2–3 tablespoons	1/3 cup
Fruits		
Canned	2–3 tablespoons	1/3 cup
Fresh	1/4–1/2 small	1/2–1 small
Juice	1/4–1/3 cup	1/2 cup
Milk Products		
Milk	1/2 cup	3/4 cup
Cheese	1/2 ounce	1 ounce
Yogurt	1/2 cup	3/4 cup
Meat, Fish, Poultry, Beans, Eggs		
Fish, poultry, meat	1/2–1 ounce	1 1/2 ounces
Dry beans	1/3 cup cooked	1/2 cup cooked
Peanut butter	1 tablespoon	1–2 tablespoons
Eggs	1/2	1

Nuts, peanuts, and seeds are not suggested for children under 4 four years of age as they may cause choking.

Eating a variety of foods helps to ensure that a variety of nutrients are available to the body. Keep encouraging your children and eat a varied diet yourself. You'll be happy with the results and be setting the stage for a lifetime of good nutrition.

Mealtimes Are a Pleasant Part of the Family Routine

To get the most benefit from family meals, mealtime should be a pleasant time. This means keeping distractions such as television, radio, and phone calls to a minimum. Turn off the TV; turn on the answering machine. Focus on the shared aspects of the meal, including pleasant conversation and positive learning. Avoid using mealtime to reprimand, scold, and bring up unpleasant aspects of the day. Avoid rushing through meals. Hurrying can lead to overeating. It takes up to 20 minutes for the brain to tell the body it is full. Eating too quickly upsets this balance and can lead to overeating.

Relax and enjoy the company of your children at the table. Often mealtime is one of the few times busy families take the time to communicate. Ask your spouse and older children questions about the activities of the day. Use this time to teach conversation and caring skills as well as reinforce appropriate eating behaviors and table manners.

Excess Juice and Sweetened Beverages Are Limited

In 1997, US consumers spent five billion dollars on refrigerated and bottled juice. Children are the single largest group of juice consumers. Fruit juice can be part of a healthy diet. If the juice is 100% juice (as opposed to "juice drinks"), a serving is considered a serving of fruit in the Food Guide Pyramid. Pediatricians used to recommend juice to increase vitamin C intake in children and as an extra source of fluids. In addition, children like juice and readily accept it, making it easy for parents to include it in their diets.

However, it is important to notice how much juice your child is drinking. Some children are drinking so much juice that it begins to replace other nutritious foods in the diet. Juices can fill the tummy, and leave the child not hungry for the variety of foods offered at meals. Drinking too much juice can result in diarrhea, excessive gas in the stomach, abdominal pain, and tooth decay. Because of these concerns, The American Academy of Pediatrics (AAP) recently released guidelines for caregivers on juice intake for kids (Table 3.3). These guidelines can help your child avoid consuming too many sugary calories, may decrease tooth decay, and will encourage more whole fruit consumption.[3]

Table 3.3 AAP Recommendations on Juice Intake for Children

Juice should not be introduced into the diets of infants before 6 months of age.
Infants should not be given juice from bottles or easily transportable covered cups that allow them to consume juice easily throughout the day. Infants should not be given juice at bedtime.
Intake of fruit juice should be limited to 4–6 ounces for children 1 to 6 years old. For children 7 to 18 years old, juice intake should be limited to 8–12 ounces or 2 servings per day.
Children should be encouraged to eat whole fruits to meet their recommended daily fruit intake.
Infants, children, and adolescents should not consume juice that is not pasteurized.
In the evaluation of children with malnutrition (overweight or underweight), the health care provider should determine the amount of juice being consumed.
In the evaluation of children with chronic diarrhea, excessive gas, stomach pain, and dental cavities, the health care provider should determine the amount of juice being consumed.
Pediatricians should routinely discuss the use of fruit juice and fruit drinks and should educate parents about differences between the two.

Table 3.4 compares the nutritional composition of whole fruits with juices. You can see that the whole fruit is a better source of fiber and vitamins than its juice counterpart.

Table 3.4 Comparing Juice and Whole Fruit

	Calories	Fiber	Vitamin A	Vitamin C
Apple, small	63	2.86 grams	5.30 RE	6.04 mg
Apple Juice, 1/2 cup	58	0.12 grams	0.12 RE	1.12 mg
Applesauce, 1/2 cup	97	1.53 grams	1.27 RE	2.17 mg
Orange, small	45	2.30 grams	20.16 RE	51.07 mg
Orange Juice, 1/2 cup	55	0.24 grams	18.68 RE	53.16 mg

Fruit Juice vs. Fruit Drinks

If you do decide to serve juice to your child, look carefully at the label. There are some important differences between fruit juice and fruit drink. To be labeled "fruit juice", the Food and Drug Administration (FDA) states that the product be "100% juice". The label on any beverage that has less than 100% juice must list the percentage of juice in the product. The terms "drink", "beverage," or "cocktail" usually indicate that there is less than 100% juice in the product. The amount of actual juice in a child's fruit drink can range from 10% juice to 99% juice. In addition, there are usually added sweeteners and flavors in these products.

Regardless of your choice, juices and sweetened beverages should be limited in the diet as recommended by the AAP. If your child is already drinking more than the guidelines recommend, you can begin decreasing the amount gradually. One way to wean a child off juice is to dilute it with water. This way they will still be getting the same quantity of liquid but you'll know they are getting fewer calories and sugar. In addition keep in mind the role you play as a model for good behaviors. Try to drink milk and water around your children rather than soda or sweet beverages. What's good for them is good for you!

Fast Food Is Limited

In our culture, it would be unrealistic for us to tell parents to completely avoid fast food. Instead, we suggest you place limits on fast-food consumption for the whole family. Fast food is very low in nutrients such as vitamin C, vitamin A, and fiber. This is primarily due to the absence of fruits and vegetables on the fast-food menu. At the same time, fast food is notoriously high in calories, fat, saturated fat, and sodium. Sadly, the marketing for fast foods is often directed at young children, with toys and prizes making the appeal very strong. If you are taking your family out for fast food once or twice a month, it is probably not much of an issue for your family. However, if you are at your local burger joint so often that the folks behind the counter know your order, it's time to set some limits for the family! Here are some tips on how to do just that.

- **Start weaning the family off fast food gradually.** Changes made abruptly (i.e. "We're never coming here again!") will be met with lots of resistance. Also if you make fast food absolutely "forbidden", it might make it even more appealing to your children. Teaching them that eating fast food in moderation is an OK thing to do occasionally is a better message than making the food forbidden and potentially more appealing. Fast-food meals should not be used as a reward and likewise the removal of fast food should not be interpreted as punishment.
- **Ask for low-fat milk or 100% juice instead of the soda and sweetened beverages.**
- **Take advantage of healthier offerings such as salad, soup, and yogurt.** The restaurants will only keep these choices on the menu if people buy them. If the prices for healthier choices seem higher, it's because there is less demand. If people were to start demanding these products, the prices would come down.
- **Consider sharing a meal with other family members.** The portions are much greater in the

super-sized meals. Order one meal and split the food. You'll save money and eat a more reasonable portion.

- **"Drive-thru" on nice days and take the meal to a park.** If you're going to eat higher calorie foods, you might as well get a little extra family activity!

Children Are Encouraged to Feed Themselves When Appropriate

An important part of feeding kids is knowing when to let them do it themselves! As soon as children are able, it's a good idea to help them serve themselves at meals. This is called "family style" dining. There are many advantages to family style dining. For starters, it helps children learn to regulate their food intake. Research has shown that children may eat up to 25% less when they serve themselves. In other words, children are usually capable of knowing how much to eat. Like the infant that knows when to stop nursing when they are full, young children retain that ability to self-regulate food.

In contrast, if the caregiver puts specific amounts of food on the plate and requires children to "clean the plate" this can lead to overeating in some children. Children may in these circumstances begin to lose the ability to identify when they are full. Giving children control over how much they eat is actually better for them in the long run. As long as you are offering a variety of nutritious food at the meal, children can decide how much of it to eat. It is quite normal for kids to eat a lot one day, and eat very little on another. Unlike adults who have pretty constant calorie needs once they stop growing, children grow in "spurts" and their calorie needs change from day to day.

Some children, especially overweight children, may be having difficulty regulating their own intake. These children may need help in understanding the feelings of fullness and hunger. This can take some time. Parents can help by keeping the mealtime relaxed and pleasant and not making a big deal about how much food the child is eating. Parents can begin to gently ask questions such as "How does your tummy feel when it is empty?" or "How does your tummy feel when it is full?" Children need to be reassured that food will be available again at another meal or snack. Sometimes when food is being restricted in some way, children will overeat whenever food *is* available because they are worried about not having access to food later.

The parents' role is vital in food regulation.

- **Keep the mealtime pleasant.**
- **Watch for cues from the child that he or she is full or perhaps not hungry at the meal.** Allow the child to say when they are full and want to stop eating.
- **Don't pressure children to clean plates.**
- **Don't make an issue if the child seems to be eating a large amount of food.**
- **Be patient and sensitive to a child's appetite.**

All Family Members, Including Children, Exercise Daily

People of all ages who are generally inactive can improve their health and well-being by becoming active. We now know that regular physical activity can substantially reduce one's risk of developing heart disease, colon cancer, diabetes, and high blood pressure. Regular exercise helps control weight, contributes to healthy bones, and reduces symptoms of anxiety and depression. Yet, more than half of all adults don't exercise regularly. Unfortunately, kids are starting to follow suit!

It is never too early to teach (and model!) the importance of regular exercise with your children. Encouraging healthy eating and physical activity in childhood can promote healthy lifestyle behaviors in children that will last a lifetime. Regular physical activity is not only an important part of staying healthy, but it's also a great way for children and parents to spend quality family time together.

Young children, however, aren't going to be too excited about aerobics classes, treadmills, or stationary bikes. Kids just want to move and have fun. Every minute that they are up moving and playing is time well spent, especially if they're having fun.

Health experts recommend that toddlers and preschoolers engage in regular physical activity that is *age* and *developmentally appropriate* (Table 3.5). Young children should not be inactive or sedentary for extended periods of time during the day. By the time children get to elementary school, the recommendations are for 30-60 minutes per day of regular physical activity. Physical activity for preschoolers must be *fun*. Children at this age are concrete thinkers. That is, they can only think in the here and now. They don't care about decreasing risk of heart disease. They want to have fun, make friends, and learn new skills. If children are enjoying the activity, there is a greater likelihood that they will continue with it. Activities should emphasize self-improvement, participation and cooperation rather than winning and losing. Avoid regimentation and offer a variety of activities. Children should be encouraged, but never forced, to participate and try new activities.

When planning physical activities, keep in mind the child's age and choose developmentally and age-appropriate activities. Most preschoolers are just learning to throw a ball overhand, kick with some precision, and balance on one foot. Focus on non-competitive games and activities that emphasize learning new skills while having fun and moving. Table 3.5 shows the developmental progress of most typical preschoolers. Activities need to be structured around these abilities.

Table 3.5 Age-Appropriate Games and Activities

Age	Walking and Running	Hopping and Jumping	Throwing and Catching	Pedaling and Steering
2–3 years	Walks more rhythmically; feet are not as widely spaced; opposite arm-leg swing. Appears hurried. Walk changes to true run.	Jumps down from step. Jumps several inches off floor with both feet, no arm action. Hops 1 to 3 times on same foot with stiff upper body and non-hopping leg held still.	Throws ball with forearm extension only; feet remain stationary. Awaits thrown ball with rigid arms outstretched.	Pushes riding toy with feet, little steering.
3–4 years	Walks up stairs, alternating feet. Walks down stairs, leading with one foot. Walks straight line.	Jumps off floor, with coordinated arm action. Broad jumps about 1 foot. Hops 4 to 6 times on same foot, flexing upper body and swinging non-hopping leg.	Throws ball with light body rotation but little or no transfer of weight with feet. Flexes elbows in preparation for catching; traps ball against chest.	Pedals and steers tricycle.
4–5 years	Walks down stairs, alternating feet. Walks circular line. Walks awkwardly on balance beam. Runs more smoothly. Gallops and ships with one foot.	Jumps upward and forward more effectively; travels greater distance. Hops 7 to 9 times on same foot; improved speed of hopping.	Throws ball with increased body rotation and some transfer of weight forward. Catches ball with hands; if unsuccessful, may still trap ball against chest.	Rides tricycle rapidly, steers smoothly.

Table 3.5 Age-Appropriate Games and Activities *(Continued)*

Age	Walking and Running	Hopping and Jumping	Throwing and Catching	Pedaling and Steering
5–6 years	Walks securely on balance beam. Increases speed of run. Gallops more smoothly. Engages in true skipping.	Jumps off floor about 1 foot. Broad jumps 3 feet. Hops 50 feet on same foot in 10 seconds. Hops with rhythmic alternation (2 hops on one foot and 2 on the other)	Has mature throwing and catching pattern. Moves arm more and steps forward during throw. Awaits thrown ball with relaxed posture, adjusting body to path and size of ball.	Rides bicycle with training wheels.

Sources: Cratty, 1986; Getchell & Roberton, 1989; Newbog, Stock, & Wnek, 1984; Roberton, 1984.

Children should be provided with an environment in which they can play and move freely and safely, both indoors and outdoors. The most important part of physical activity is that it is enjoyable. The second most important part is that the whole family is taking part in the fun! Have some fun with your kids! Go to a park or playground. Walk there if it isn't too far. Instead of watching the kids play, join in the fun. Play tag, push them on the swings, play hide and seek! You can benefit from the extra exercise yourself! Plan active outdoor vacations like beach and camping trips.

Television/Computer/Video Game Time Is Limited for All Family Members

We are seeing a decrease in regular physical activity in both kids and adults. At the same time, we're seeing a huge increase in time spent being inactive, that is, watching TV and playing video and computer games. Even very young children such as toddlers and preschoolers are spending hours each day in front of the television and the computer. Even though the computer may seem a little more educational and interactive than TV, it is still a sedentary activity.

It is the parents' absolute responsibility to turn the TV off. Kids may complain at first, but they will eventually find something else to do. Even playing with blocks or making puzzles is more active than television viewing. Better still would be using the "TV off" time for engaging in some fun physical activity for the whole family. Even on a rainy day or a day when you must stay indoors, put some music on and dance around the room or have a parade. Kids will love it! They will be happy spending time with you.

Parents Serve as Role Models for Healthy Eating and Regular Physical Activity

You can offer your child nutritious food and throw away your television, but no significant impact will be made if you, the caregiver, aren't modeling the behaviors you hope to change in your children.

You can't tell your child to limit sweetened beverages if you're drinking soda in front of them! You can't tell a child, "No TV!" while you sit for hours watching the news and endless hours of reality TV. You can't tell your child "Go play!" when you haven't moved a muscle yet this year!

Kids of all ages, but especially little ones, are like sponges, soaking up everything we give them. Model the behavior you want to see and you will begin to see that behavior.

Special Situations

You may not always be in control of the type of food your child is getting or the environment in which he or she is being fed. This is especially true if your child is in some type of day-care setting. If this is the case, you can still be an important advocate for your child's health by choosing a center or child-care situation that has nutrition and physical activity standards similar to your own. To find this out, you need to ask the right questions. The following sections feature some nutrition and feeding-related questions to keep in mind when you are choosing a child-care setting.

Nutrition Considerations in Child-Care Settings

For infants:

Does the center allow you to bring in pumped breast milk and/or allow you to visit and breastfeed your baby whenever you can?

Does the center have a safe place to store your labeled bottles (i.e. refrigerator with sufficient space)?

Does the center feed the babies on demand? This is preferable to feeding on a schedule set by the staff at the center.

Does the center allow the baby to decide when he/she is full or do they force the child to finish the bottle?

For toddlers and preschoolers:

Does the center participate in the Child and Adult Care Food Program? (See Appendix 5 for more information on this and other related organizations.) If they do, then you know that appropriate nutrition standards are in place for all foods served there. If not, you may want to encourage the center to participate in the program.

Are children encouraged to feed themselves?

Are meals and snacks appropriate for their age and developmental ability?

Is milk offered with lunch and juice limited to four ounces per day?

Does the center give you a detailed description of what your child ate during the day at your request?

Physical Activity Considerations in Child-Care Settings

Quality day-care centers have very limited or no television access for the children. In addition, a good center has a curriculum that includes lots of opportunity throughout the day for kids to move and play. As mentioned earlier in this chapter, activities should be age and developmentally appropriate with an emphasis on fun and not on competition. If you are not sure of your center's policy on television and physical activity time, you need to ask the director. He or she should have a specific policy in place and be willing to discuss it with you. Examine playground equipment at the center carefully. Make sure the equipment is age and developmentally appropriate and kept in good repair.

If your child is in a family day-care home, then you need to share your feelings about nutrition and physical activity with your day-care provider. Find out how much television, computer, and other sedentary activities are allowed during the day. Notice if there is a safe place for kids to play outdoors.

Staying on the Right Track

Making healthy lifestyle changes when the children are young is ideal. At this point in their development, children are most able to accept the changes and incorporate them permanently into their lives and yours. However, changes need to begin small and grow gradually in order for them to be permanent. If necessary, focus on just one of the Top Ten Healthy Behaviors for your young child.

Decide what improvements you wish to make and work on them, one step at a time. Once you have success with one behavior change, you will then feel capable of moving on to another behavior that needs improvement. Something as simple as reducing juice intake or deciding to take family walks each night can be great steps towards a healthier family. All changes, no matter how small, are significant. Your family will benefit and feel great.

If you have older children, check out the next two chapters, which emphasize the unique needs of school-agers and teenagers. If not, you may still want to read them now and bookmark them for later because your kids will soon be there! Now may also be a good time to check out some of the menu planning and recipes in later chapters to find easy meals and cooking ideas for your busy family.

> Now, back to Anna and her mother–you will recall that we left them stranded at the table! Anna's behavior is really quite normal for a child her age. As long as she is growing well and is healthy, Mom needs to relax. Looking at the stages of development in Table 3.1, we see that the best reaction from Mom is to respect Anna's ability to dislike or like a new food. Scolding and bribing will only encourage Anna to dig in her heels even more. The parent's responsibility is to continue to offer a healthy and varied diet. As long as Anna is developmentally on track for her age, Mom needs to wait out this "food jag." Anna will eat!

Sources:

1. Ogden, C., Flegal, K., Carroll, M., & Johnson, C. (2000). Prevalence and trends in overweight among US children and adolescents. *Journal of the American Medical Association,* 288, 1728–1732.
2. Stockmyer, C. (2001). Remember when mom wanted you home for dinner? *Nutrition Reviews,* 59, No. 2, 57–60.
3. American Academy of Pediatrics Policy Statement: The use and misuse of fruit juice in pediatrics. (2001). *Pediatrics,* 107, 1210–1213.

CHAPTER 4

Creating a Healthy Environment for Your School-Aged Child

Maggie is in fourth grade. She has always been a little chubby. Lately some of the kids at school have been teasing her and calling her "fat." Maggie is feeling really upset and embarrassed about this. In gym class, she can't keep up with the other kids. She starts to breathe heavily and her face turns red when she exercises. Maggie's mom was chubby as a kid, too, but she is now normal weight and works out daily at the gym at her office. Maggie's dad has never had a weight problem, but is very conscious of keeping fit. He, too, works out regularly at the gym while Maggie is at school. Mom and Dad are concerned about Maggie. They've been buying her special "diet" foods and nagging her to stop watching so much TV. Are they on the right path? What else can they do?

Your School-Ager and Food

As soon as your children set off for school, you are losing a little of them to their newfound independence. It's an exciting time, though it can be a bit frightening, too! For several hours a day, you are no longer in control of their activities, including their food choices. The wonderful part about this is the exciting exposure they will have to a wide range of new friends, new cultures, and new foods.

Even if they bring their lunch from home, there will be lots of new food for them to see. Their friends will bring different items and the school will serve new things as well. They may come home and urge you to buy foods that the other kids have in their lunches. Some of these will be healthy new foods and others will be the foods you may have been limiting in your home. You'll need to find the right balance when feeding your school-ager. If you try to control their eating too much, they may end up with some unhealthy eating behaviors, such as sneaking food, spending lunch/milk money on unhealthy snacks, or compulsive overeating.

In addition to new foods, your child will be exposed to and be more aware of the different body types that children have. As we discussed in Chapter 1, children grow and develop differently. Puberty for some children will begin as soon as age nine or ten. It's important at this time to teach them about acceptance of others' differences, especially with regard to body size. They need to know what to expect from their own bodies and to respect themselves and others for who they are. Encouraging them to eat well and be physically active will help them to appreciate their bodies, regardless of their size.

This chapter will focus on the special needs of school-aged children. The emphasis will be on helping children to make healthy food choices and to include regular physical activity in their lives in a fun, safe, and noncompetitive environment. As always, we'll also emphasize the importance of the parents in modeling and supporting healthy behaviors and attitudes.

Top Ten Healthy Behaviors

The following list features behaviors that we feel can make all the difference as you help your child make the daily decisions about food and activity that will lead to healthy lifestyle behaviors.

1. Children eat a healthy breakfast every day.
2. Children eat a healthy lunch at school, and parents are informed about lunch choices at school.
3. Children choose healthy snacks.
4. Children drink non-fat (skim) or low-fat (1%) milk.
5. Sweetened beverages are limited.
6. Fast food is limited.
7. Children get at least 60 minutes per day of physical activity.
8. Sedentary activities are limited.
9. Parents model healthy eating and exercise habits.
10. Parents emphasize the importance of a healthy body image for children.

Children Eat a Healthy Breakfast

Start the day right; eat breakfast! One of the easiest ways to improve your child's health, attention span, and academic performance is to make sure they eat breakfast. Children and adults who eat breakfast eat better throughout the day and usually regulate their weight better than those who don't eat breakfast. See Table 4.1 for more details on how eating breakfast helps kids do better in school. Eating breakfast "jump starts" the metabolism, fueling the body to be ready for the activities of the day. Without breakfast, children tend to have trouble focusing at school, are inattentive, and may even display behavior problems.

Table 4.1 Why Breakfast Helps

Kids Who Eat Breakfast Learn Better
Concentrate better
Make fewer errors
Score higher on tests
Are more creative
Work faster

Table 4.1 Why Breakfast Helps *(Continued)*

Kids Who Eat Breakfast Behave Better in School
Cause fewer fights
Are more cooperative
Are less likely to be sent to principal's office for discipline problems
Get along better with classmates

Source: USDA. (1994–96) Continuing Survey of Food Intake by Individuals.

Despite the well-documented benefits of eating breakfast, up to 16% of children aged 6–18 skip breakfast on a regular basis. Girls are more likely to skip breakfast than boys. This is usually because girls are trying to reduce their daily calorie intake. Other reasons for skipping breakfast are lack of time, lack of available food, or the absence of an adult to supervise the morning routine.

If time is the problem, you need to make breakfast a bigger priority in your family's lives. This may mean getting up a few minutes earlier. You can set the table and put out some breakfast items the night before to save time in a busy morning routine. Breakfast can be a great family meal to start the day. For some families, this is a good time to chat about the upcoming day. If you really don't have any time in the morning or someone can't be home to get breakfast going for the kids, then you may want to find out if your school has a breakfast program. School breakfast programs can be nutritious, inexpensive, and convenient for busy working parents.

What Is a Healthy Breakfast?

A healthy breakfast has servings from at least three food groups from the Food Guide Pyramid. For example, breakfast should contain a fruit or fruit juice, bread or cereal (preferably whole grain), and low-fat or non-fat milk. A healthy breakfast could consist of a whole grain cereal with milk and a glass of juice. Try to avoid serving too many sugary foods at breakfast on a regular basis, such as sweetened fruit drinks, soda, or fruit-filled pastries. A breakfast too high in sugar can cause a quick rise in blood sugar and energy in children followed by a rapid energy drop about an hour later that leaves the child feeling hungry again.

Whatever your choice, breakfast should be filling enough to last until the next scheduled meal or snack. For some children, that may be just a few hours but for others, it may be more than four hours. Find out when your child eats lunch at school and what time snacks, if any, are allowed. This will help you decide how much food your child needs for breakfast.

If your child isn't typically hungry in the morning, they should at least have a glass of juice and a breakfast bar to munch on the way out the door or on the bus. While including three food groups is a great idea, it isn't always possible. *Any* breakfast is better than no breakfast! For more quick breakfast ideas, see Chapter 7. Don't forget to eat breakfast yourself! Remember that children model the behavior they see. Eat a healthy breakfast with your kids and they will do the same.

Children Eat a Healthy Lunch

What's for lunch? Now that we've established a routine for a healthy breakfast, let's talk about lunch.

Lunch at school is a time for fun and conversation at the table as well as for eating. These days kids are often rushed at lunch as the lunch period continues to get shorter to allow for more academic contact hours. Your child needs a quick nutritious lunch that will carry him or her through the afternoon.

Bag vs. School Lunch?

Whether you choose to have your child bring lunch from home or buy it at school is really a personal decision. Packing a bag lunch is not necessarily healthier than school lunch if you aren't careful about what goes in the bag. Some studies have shown that children get more nutrients by eating what the school provides than by packing a lunch. Part of the problem is that many children pack their own lunches with prepackaged chips, fruit snacks, sweetened beverages, and desserts. It is great to have children get involved in food preparation and pack their own lunches but make sure that you are in charge of providing them with healthy choices when they do so.

A healthy lunch with maximum staying power and nutrition has a source of protein (peanut butter, lean deli meat, egg, or cheese), a source of bread or grains (preferably whole grain), a fruit and/or vegetable serving, and a beverage, preferably low-fat milk. Usually milk can be purchased at school and is a convenient source of high quality protein, calcium and other vitamins and minerals. If you choose to pack a beverage for your child, choose 100% fruit juice or water, if possible. Look at the label on the fruit juice packs or boxes to see if the juice is labeled "100% juice" or "juice drink." The "juice drink" may be no more than water, sugar, and fruit flavoring. Don't forget to pack an ice pack to keep food safe to eat until lunchtime!

School lunch can be a nutritious and convenient option for many kids. Find out if your school participates in the National School Lunch Program. If so, then there are specific nutrition standards that will be met for lunch. For example, lunch must meet one third of the calorie needs of the child. It must, over the course of the week, have no more than 30% of calories from fat, no more than 10% of calories from saturated fat, and be a good source of vitamins A and C. This usually means that fruits and vegetables are part of the meal. Some schools are better at meeting these guidelines than others are. If you're not sure, why not take a little time and enjoy a meal at school with your child. You'll see firsthand what's being served.

Watch out for a la carte options! This is when kids spend their lunch money on extra items instead of buying the featured meal. Often these a la carte items are snack items high in fat, calories, sugar, and sodium, such as French fries, sweetened beverages, chips, ice cream and cookies. These foods can certainly be allowed occasionally as part of a healthy diet, but really shouldn't be a child's mainstay for lunch.

Regardless of whether your child brings lunch or buys it at school, they need an environment at school that is conducive to healthy eating. The United States Department of Agriculture recently highlighted a few questions to ask schools about the nutrition environment. The emphasis is on children having a comfortable place to eat, enough time to eat and healthy choices available to them. This atmosphere is best suited for all children in the cafeteria and encourages children to eat well.

Table 4.2 Evaluating the School Nutrition Environment

Ask the following questions to assess the nutrition environment in your child's school:
Do students have a comfortable place to sit and eat lunch?
Do they have enough time to eat?
Is the lunch period too early? Too late?
Does the school teach good nutrition in the classroom – and then sell soda to raise money?
Are healthy food choices available at school parties and after-school activities as well as in the school dining room?
Does the school offer school breakfast only during exam week?

Check into your school's cafeteria situation. Ask questions (see the examples in Table 4.2). If you are not happy with the answers, get involved! You may find there are plenty of other parents with similar concerns. Start small and choose one or two concerns at first. Involve as many influential folks as you can (e.g., the principal, school food service director, teachers, parents, school nurses). It's never too late to make a change!

Children Choose Healthy Snacks

Snack Attack! Contrary to what some think, snacking does have a role as part of a healthy diet. Many people, when they think of snacking, think exclusively of candy, chips, and sweetened beverages. Healthy snacking, however, can be an important element of a healthy diet. Some children must go many hours between meals and snacking can help fill the gap. Snacks, if chosen wisely, can complement the nutrition for the day instead of detracting from it. You can use snack time as a way to introduce fruits and vegetables to a hungry child. See Table 4.3 for healthy snacking tips.

Table 4.3 Snacking Dos and Don'ts

Do serve snacks at scheduled times, emphasizing nutritious foods from the Food Guide Pyramid.
Do keep snacks small enough so children are not too full to eat the next meal.
Do offer snacks far enough from meals so children are not too full to eat the next meal.
Do serve food from at least two different food groups at a snack break (i.e., string cheese and pretzels).
Do keep cut up fresh fruit and vegetables on hand and ready for a quick nutritious snack.
Do keep a supply of quick snacks such as cereal, pretzels, nuts, low-fat granola bars, and dried fruit available.
Do keep the healthy snack options in plain view so children will see them first and grab them.
Do strive for portion control. Instead of serving from the big bag of chips, portion out snacks into individual portions for serving or purchase the snack size.

Don't serve dessert for snacks.
Don't serve snacks too close to a meal.
Don't serve snacks randomly throughout the day (i.e. no "grazing").
Don't serve sweetened beverages, such as soda and sweetened sports drinks, for snacks. (These drinks fill tummies while supplying few if any nutrients).
Don't get carried away buying lots of "reduced fat" or "sugar free" products for snacks. (Children and adults have not been shown to benefit from these products and often end up eating larger portions and more calories thinking these are somehow healthier than the original product.)

Children Drink Non-Fat (Skim) or Low-Fat (1%) Milk

Milk is a good source of high quality protein, calcium, and many vitamins and minerals. A glass of 1% or non-fat milk has about the same number of calories as a glass of soda. However, all the soda contains is sugar! Milk is a nutritional bargain. There is no nutritional difference between whole milk and non-fat. There is simply less fat and therefore, fewer calories in the non-fat variety. Healthy children over the age of two don't need to drink whole milk. Even reduced fat (2%) milk has quite a few more calories than 1% or non-fat. Work with your family to get everyone drinking 1% or non-fat milk.

The Food Guide Pyramid recommends 2–3 servings per day from the milk group. If your child has milk on breakfast cereal, milk with lunch at school, and a glass of milk at dinner, they have met the recommendations. If your child cannot drink milk due to allergies, intolerances, or religious/cultural reasons, you should consider fortified soy milk as an alternative. Soy milk does not provide the exact same nutrition as cow's milk, but if it is fortified, it can be similar. Be sure whatever milk alternative you choose has calcium. Children need calcium for strong bone growth and development. Unfortunately, as children get older, they seem to get less and less of the calcium they need. This is especially true for girls. Figure 4.1 shows how calcium intake generally decreases as children get older.

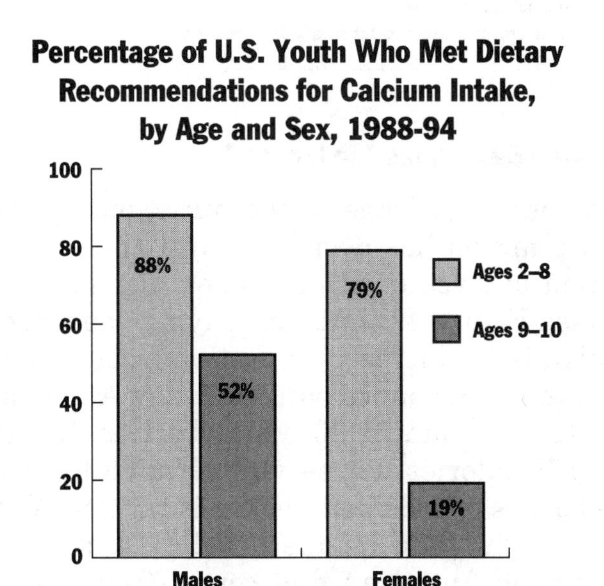

Figure 4.1 Percentage of U.S. Youth Who Met Dietary Recommendations for Calcium Intake, by Age and Sex, 1988–94

The best source of calcium in our diets comes from dairy products such as milk, yogurt, and cheese. Some vegetables, such as spinach, contain natural calcium, too. However, the body is not as good at absorbing some of these sources of calcium. The body very easily absorbs the calcium in dairy products. Recently, new products have become available that have calcium added to them. These include orange juice with calcium and cereals with added calcium. The calcium in these products is generally easy for the body to absorb. For people who don't drink very much milk, these products might be a good addition to your diet. Table 4.4 shows some more easy ways to increase your family's intake of calcium.

Table 4.4 More Calcium for Your Family

Try making smoothies with the kids (See Chapter 8 for recipe ideas).
Have kids buy non-fat milk instead of soda or sweetened drinks with lunch.
Offer yogurt or frozen yogurt for a snack.
Offer kids cheese and crackers for a snack.
Offer a pudding or an ice cream dessert to satisfy a kid's sweet tooth.

Sweetened Beverages Are Limited

Despite our knowledge of the nutritional power in milk, its consumption has decreased over the years while consumption of sweetened beverages like soda has steadily risen (see Figure 4.2). Accompanying the increase in consumption is an increase in portion sizes. Years ago, soda was served in 6.5 ounce bottles. Today, Americans are normally served soda in 20 ounce bottles. That's an additional 178 calories per serving! If a child drinks five 20 ounce bottles of soda per week this can translate into a 12 pound weight gain in one year! In fact, 37% of added sugar in the American diet comes from soft drinks and other sweetened beverages.[1] Fifty-six percent of eight-year old children drink soda every day! Given the fact that there is no nutritional value to soda, this is very dis-

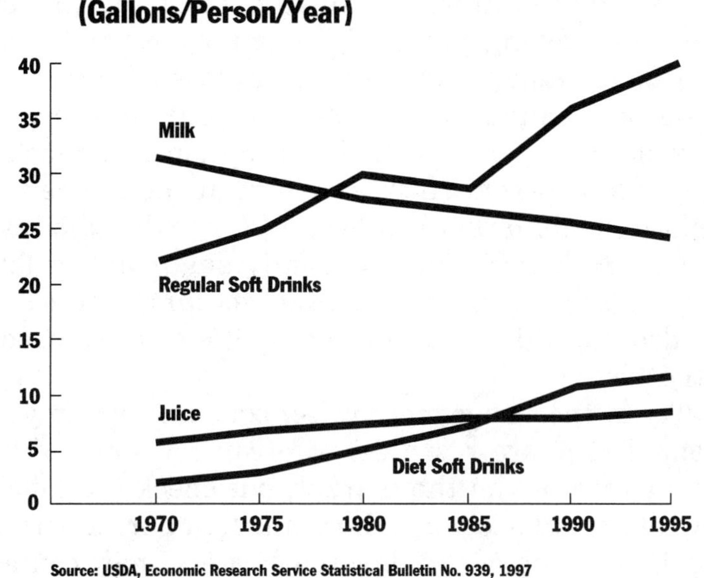

Figure 4.2 Beverages Available in the U.S. Food Supply (Gallons/Person/Year)

turbing. For the same number of calories as soda, a child could get substantially greater nutrition from a healthier beverage. As you can see in Table 4.5, sweetened beverages have little or no nutritional value to offer when compared to a glass of 100% orange juice or low-fat milk.

Table 4.5 Comparing Beverages Choices

	Non-Diet Soda	Sports Drink+	Orange Juice	1% Milk
Calories	153	90	164	153
Sugar, g	39	23	37*	18*
Vitamin A, RE	0	0	56	216
Vitamin C, mg	0	0	160	4
Calcuim, mg	0	0	37	450
Potassium, mg	0	40	710	571

*The sugar in orange juice is fructose, a naturally occuring fruit sugar and the sugar in milk is naturally occurring lactose.

+Most sports drinks come in larger than 12 oz. containers.

What about Sports Drinks?

If your child is in for an all-day soccer tournament and will be sweating profusely, you may want to consider offering sports drinks. However, unless your child is exercising continuously for over an hour or exercising in extreme heat, water is the best option to quench thirst. Most people exercising less than an hour need only to replace the fluid that has been lost, not the calories. What sports drinks offer is essentially sugar and a few electrolytes such as potassium and sodium. The calories in the drink could end up exceeding the calories used in the activity!

Try to encourage more water consumption in your children. If they are resistant, you can try some of the new flavored waters on the market, but check the label to see how many calories (and how much sugar) are in a serving. Even some of the flavored "waters" now contain considerable calories.

Fast Food Is Limited

As we mentioned in the last chapter, in our culture it would be unrealistic for us to tell parents to completely avoid fast food. Limiting fast-food consumption for the whole family is a worthy goal however. Fast food is notoriously low in nutrients and notoriously high in calories, fat, saturated fat, and sodium. Since fast-food marketing is often deliberately aimed at children (toys, movie tie-ins, cartoon "spokespeople," etc.) it is hard to avoid but the following tips should help you reduce the role it plays in your family's lifestyle. You may also want to review Chapter 3 for more detailed information on the hazards of fast food.

- **Start weaning the family off fast food gradually.** Changes made abruptly (i.e., "We're never coming here again!") will be met with lots of resistance.

- **Order low-fat milk or 100% juice instead of the soda and sweetened beverages.**
- **Take advantage of healthier offerings such as salad, soup, and yogurt.**
- **Consider sharing a meal with other family members.** Order one adult meal and split the food. You'll save money and eat a more reasonable portion.
- **"Drive-thru" on nice days and take the meal to a park.** Combine your less-than-healthy meal with some very healthy outdoor activity!
- **Choose your entrée carefully.** Chicken and fish are not always the best choices. We tend to think poultry and fish are better for us than red meat. Not necessarily! Fast-food restaurants often bread and fry chicken or fish. The end product can have as much *or more fat* and calories than a hamburger. Choose chicken or fish that is broiled, baked, or grilled. If you're not sure how an entree is prepared, go ahead and ask. Most fast food restaurants will provide nutritional data for their menu items. See Table 4.6 for more comparison information on various popular fast-food choices. You might be surprised at how the burger compares to the non-red meat choices. Keep in mind however that this data is for a regular hamburger not a super-sized double-patty specialty burger option.
- **Order a side salad instead of fries.** It's a great way to increase your vegetable intake. Some restaurants even offer "shaker" salads packed in convenient containers, making them easier to eat on the go! Just beware of the hidden calories and fat in the salad dressings. Two ounces of ranch dressing (about one of those packets) provides 20 grams of

fat! That's as much fat as a Quarter Pounder! Opt for "lite" or reduced-fat dressings or use less of the heavier ones.

Table 4.6 Comparing Fast-Food Choices

Fast-Food Item	Grams of Fat	Calories per Serving
Burger King Chicken Sandwich	36	685
McDonalds Filet-O-Fish	24	370
KFC Colonel's Chicken Sandwich	24	482
Taco Bell Chicken Burrito	12	334
McDonalds Regular Hamburger	8	255

Children Get at Least 60 Minutes Per Day of Physical Activity

Regular physical activity strengthens bones and the heart while building strong muscles. Research shows us it even helps students perform better in school. A 2001 study from the California Department of Education found that students with a higher fitness level scored better on academic achievement tests than those students who were less fit.[2] Unfortunately, most kids are not getting anywhere near the recommended amount. Nearly 50% of young people ages 12–21 do not engage in physical activity on a regular basis. As children get older, their level of physical activity decreases still more. Our increasingly technological society is an increasingly sedentary society.

Healthy children are encouraged to get at least 60 minutes per day of physical activity. This activity doesn't have to occur all at once. Activities done in 10-minute increments or more throughout the day count towards the daily goal. The activities also don't need to involve competitive sports. At this age, children definitely want to be having fun while they're moving. It is likely that any activity that is enjoyable will be done by children for longer periods of time. If they find the activity rote or boring (i.e., treadmills or calisthenics!), they will quickly look for ways to get out of it. In addition, if they are sensitive about their athletic abilities, they may shy away from sports. Involve them in something fun that promotes physical activity without competition like bike riding or hiking.

Figure 4.3 shows the government's Physical Activity Pyramid for kids. You can see it is shaped like the Food Guide Pyramid. The graphic places more emphasis on the larger piece of the pyramid (playing outside), and less emphasis on the tip of the pyramid (sitting and watching television). What is also notable about the Activity Pyramid is the focus on family activities such as going for a walk, riding bikes, playing at the park and swimming together.

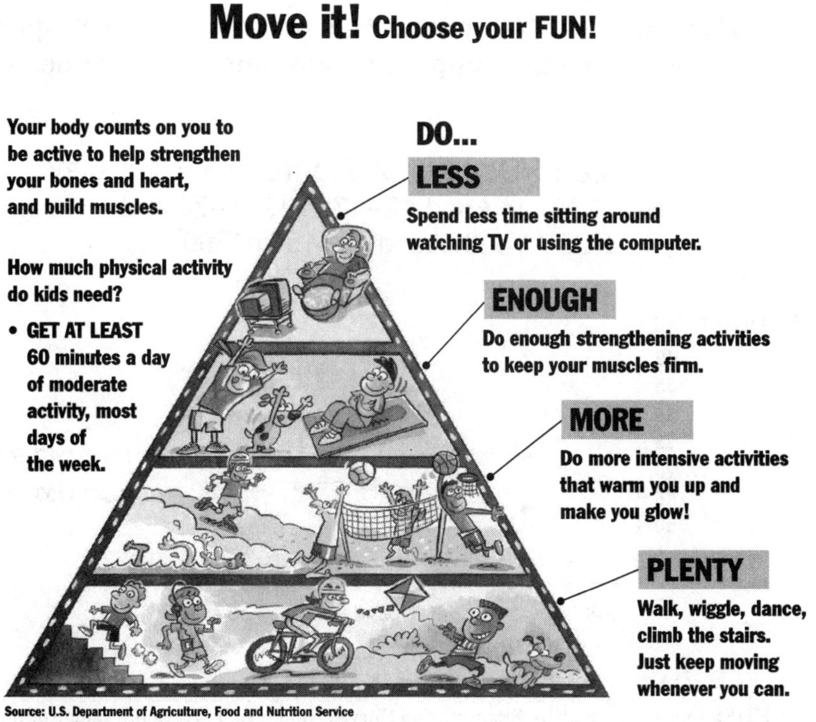

Move it! Choose your FUN!
Your body counts on you to be active to help strengthen your bones and heart, and build muscles.
How much physical activity do kids need?
• GET AT LEAST 60 minutes a day of moderate activity, most days of the week.
DO...
LESS
Spend less time sitting around watching TV or using the computer.
ENOUGH
Do enough strengthening activities to keep your muscles firm.
MORE
Do more intensive activities that warm you up and make you glow!
PLENTY
Walk, wiggle, dance, climb the stairs. Just keep moving whenever you can.
Source: U.S. Department of Agriculture, Food and Nutrition Service

Figure 4.3 Move it! Choose your fun!

Sedentary Activities Are Limited

Naturally, since we're encouraging increased physical activity, sedentary activities must correspondingly be limited. As kids begin to sit around less, they will ultimately be moving more, as the Physical Activity Pyramid recommends. However, it can be difficult, in this age of increased television, computer, and video game usage, to get kids to turn the electronics off! In 1970, only 6% of children lived in homes with three or more TVs. By 1999, 60% of children lived in homes with three or more TVs. And 77% of sixth graders have a TV in their bedroom!

It's time to become aware of exactly how much time your child is spending on these sedentary activities. Figure 4.4 clearly shows the frightening correlation between television viewing and obesity. As television-viewing time increases, obesity rates increase.

Parents need to monitor the situation and set specific limits on TV time, computer time, and video game time.

Prevalence of Obesity by Hours of TV per Day
NHES Youth Aged 12–17 in 1967–70 and
NLSY Youth Aged 10–15 in 1990*

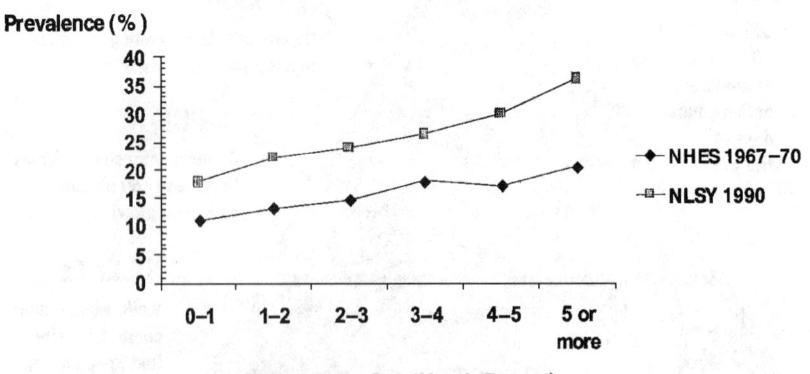

* NHES (National Healthy Examination Survey) and NLSY (National Longitudinal Survey of Youth)

Figure 4.4 Prevalence of Obesity by Hours of TV Viewed per Day 1967–70 and 1990

Many families make an effort to have "TV turnoff day." You may want to set aside one day of the week to do this. You'll need to make that day fun, however, with an extra emphasis on family fun and physical activity so the kids will look forward to such days and even request more! It also helps to involve other families in your community with this effort. There's strength in numbers. If your child's friends have similar restrictions on TV viewing, they can find things to do together when the TV is off! If your community doesn't recognize "TV Turnoff Week," you can check out this national organization on-line and consider starting a local effort. Visit www.tvturnoff.org for more information.

Parents Model Healthy Eating and Exercise Habits

If you're still not seeing changes in your child's eating habits and physical activity, you may want to look more closely at your own. Parents cannot expect certain behaviors from their kids without modeling those behaviors themselves. In other words, don't just "talk the talk," be sure to "walk the walk"!

Families play a critical role in shaping a child's physical activity experience. Motivation to become active starts at home. Studies have found that children will be more active if their parents and siblings are. Children also tend to be more physically active in homes where the parents support the activities that children choose.

Changes in eating and physical activity need to be family-centered. It's great if you go to the gym on your lunch hour, but that's not a behavior that your child is actually seeing. Go to the gym, but also come home and suggest a family walk after dinner. Don't own a bike? Consider buying, renting, or getting a used one. Stock the fridge with healthy snacks for everyone in the family, not just for the kids.

Here are a few tips for parents on increasing physical activity for their families. This list is adapted from the USDA's "Ten Steps for Parents; Making Physical Activity Easy."

- Create safe places for kids to play. *Watch over children's activities.*
- Set a good example. *Be active with your children.*
- Promote physical activity. *Encourage children to be physically active at home, at school, and with friends.*
- Limit sitting-around time. *Alternate time spent sitting with time spent moving.*
- Establish an active routine. *Set aside time each day as activity time.*
- Coach a team. *Encourage children to participate in school and community sports.*
- Throw an activity party. *Make your child's birthday party activity-centered (Host it at the public pool, at the park, or at a local Y.)*
- Work with your school. *Be sure your child's school offers physical activity time for all students.*
- Incorporate physical activity in your daily life. *Use the stairs instead of the elevator; walk or ride a bike instead of driving a car.*
- Involve children in family chores like raking leaves or walking the dog. *Chores like vacuuming, mopping, and dusting can also be quite a work out.*
- Set limits on the amount of time children spend watching television and playing video or computer games. *Limit to a maximum of two hours per day.*
- For every hour children participate in a sedentary activity (e.g., watching television or playing computer games), encourage them to take a 10-minute physical activity break.

- Plan and participate in family activities that involve physical activity. Visit a new park, hike a trail, bike, rollerblade, sled, ski, or just play outside.

Parents Emphasize the Importance of a Healthy Body Image for Children

We strongly emphasize the importance of promoting and role-modeling healthy eating and physical fitness. This emphasis is very different from an emphasis on losing weight and watching the scale. In fact, your best response to an overweight child is *not* to make an issue of the weight itself. Focus your energy on encouraging healthy lifestyle habits instead. Research has shown that restrictive dieting is not only unhealthy for children it also is not effective in changing behavior or weight.

The most effective approach is the family-centered approach to fitness and a healthy lifestyle. Kids don't want to feel singled out and the emotional and social toll of being overweight is already very significant without added parental pressure. Children with a poor body image are more depressed and overall have a poor quality of life. Your responsibility is to teach your child the importance of a healthy, active lifestyle. Let your pediatrician evaluate their growth and development. Don't forget that children have very different patterns of growth.

In Chapter 3, we discussed the importance of knowing your child's developmental stage as it relates to eating behaviors. Table 4.7 shows the developmental stage for the school-aged group and the related eating behaviors. These stages were identified by noted psychologist Eric Erikson and adapted by Drs. Laurel Branen and Joanne Fletcher, leading nutrition experts from the University of Idaho. You may find these strategies useful to keep in mind when making decisions about your children's food intake.

Table 4.7 Fletcher and Branen's Adaptation of Erikson's Psychosocial Stages Application for Children's Eating Skills Development

Age: MIDDLE CHILDHOOD
STAGE: INDUSTRY VERSUS INFERIORITY Children develop feelings that they can make things, a sense of "I am capable."

Age: MIDDLE CHILDHOOD
FEEDING BEHAVIORS
INDUSTRY
Child discerns when he or she is hungry or full and acts on these cues.
Environment is set so the children can make their snacks or simple meals.
Children choose menus for meals.
Children make suggestions for trying new foods.
Children prepare foods for sharing with friends.
Children help set schedules for mealtimes.
INFERIORITY (Avoid these strategies!)
Children's plates are pre-served.
Adult admonishes and demeans child's attempts at making or serving food.
Children are required to clean their plates.
Children are required to taste everything at the mealtime.

Since we're talking about growing, the next chapter looks at those ever-growing, constantly eating teens! If you're ready to think about the issues surrounding teenagers, you will want to go ahead to Chapter 5.

In conclusion, let's get back to Maggie. She is struggling with her body image right now. It's not uncommon for children around this age to gain some extra body fat in preparation for an upcoming growth spurt. Her parents would do well to relax a little about her weight and focus on improving a positive body image and self-esteem. Promoting healthy eating and fitness for the whole family can be an effective way to do this. Rather than buying Maggie "special" foods, Maggie needs to be eating the same foods as everyone in the family, i.e. healthy food. She needs to be involved in the menu planning and be given some choices about nutritious foods. Her parents also need to include more physical activity as a family activity. It's terrific that Mom and Dad are both working at being fit, but Maggie needs to be exercising and having fun with them. Maggie will feel better about her body when she sees how strong and fit she can be. Unfortunately, there is usually not enough activity time in school, so Maggie's parents need to find ways to increase her level of fitness with some activities outside of school.

Hopefully, with the emphasis away from the shame of being overweight, Maggie will focus her energies on becoming a strong, healthy and active child. This will likely result in permanent lifestyle changes that will allow her to gradually grow into an appropriate weight for her age.

Sources:

1. Guthrie, J.F. and Morton, J.F. (2000). Sources of added sweeteners in the diets of Americans. *Journal of the American Dietetic Association,* 100, 43–48.
2. California Department of Education. (2002). State study proves physically fit kids perform better academically. News Release #02-37. Retrieved May 27, 2003, from http://www.cde.ca.gov/news/releases2002/rel37.

CHAPTER 5

Creating a Healthy Environment for Your Teenager

Martin is a 14-year-old overweight boy who gets home from school at 3 p.m. Famished, he grabs the open bag of chips in the cabinet and quickly polishes it off. He's thirsty so he goes for a cold soda from the fridge. He then sits in front of the TV and plays video games until Mom and Dad get home from work at 6:30. Dinner won't be ready until 7:30, so Martin munches on cheese and crackers until then. What can Martin's parents do to encourage some healthier behaviors?

Your Teenager and Food

Today's teens are the masters of multi-tasking! They go to school, play sports, have part-time jobs, are responsible for chores at home, and often have very busy social schedules. All of these responsibilities leave little time to attend to their nutrition and physical activity habits. Their demanding schedules combined with their increased independence can result in a steady diet of convenience foods. From vending machines to fast food restaurants and coffee shop pick-me-ups, many teens are consuming a diet quite low in nutritional value. Yet, important physical, cognitive, social, and emotional changes are occurring during the teen years. Teens will acquire 15–20% of their height, 50% of their adult weight, and 45% of their total skeletal mass during these years. Consequently, their nutritional needs are very high.

On the other hand, obesity rates among teenagers are at an all-time high, with over 15% of teens falling into the overweight category.[1] And overweight teens are very likely to stay overweight as they become adults. A teenager with a BMI-for-age in the 60th percentile or greater has a 36% chance of being overweight when he becomes an adult.[2] The teen years are also a time in life when great emphasis is placed on appearances. Overweight teens are more likely to be depressed and suffer from low self-esteem compared to their normal-weight peers. Teens often attempt dieting unsuccessfully as social pressures build. These diets are often in conflict with healthy eating habits and do not include an emphasis on increased physical activity. Eating disorders are frequently diagnosed in this age group as many teens try unhealthy and dangerous approaches to weight loss.

Once they become teens, children are increasingly making their own food choices, using their own money, and are no longer under the watchful eyes of Mom or Dad. They have more choices available to them than ever. Teen food choices are more influenced by factors such as peer pressure, social events, time, money, convenience, and taste than they are by their parents. Parents get understandably frustrated with this situation, feeling as if they have little or no control.

However, the picture needn't be as bleak as it sounds. Kids in this age group need to feel they are in control. They often are willing to make changes if they see the immediate value to these changes. If they have a desire to change and a supportive environment to make changes, they can improve their nutritional status while maintaining the control they seek.

This chapter will focus on the special needs of teenagers. The emphasis will be on the critical role of parents in helping their teens to make better choices about nutrition and physical activity.

Top Ten Healthy Behaviors

The following list features behaviors that we feel can make all the difference as you help your teenager make the daily decisions about food and activity that will lead to healthy lifestyle behaviors.

1. Teens eat breakfast regularly.
2. Teens make healthy meal choices at home and away from home.
3. Parents emphasize the importance of family mealtime.
4. Teens make healthy snack choices.
5. Teens choose healthy beverages.
6. Teens don't skip meals.
7. Overweight teens are encouraged to make healthy decisions about diets.
8. Regular physical activity is encouraged.
9. A healthy body image is encouraged and supported.
10. Parents support the decisions their teenagers make about nutrition and physical activity.

Teens Eat Breakfast Regularly

One of the worst nutrition decisions anyone can make is skipping breakfast. Unfortunately, it's also one of the most common mistakes teenagers make! Thirty-five percent of teenage girls skip breakfast daily and 50% of kids aged 9–15 skip breakfast at least once per week.[3] As we discussed in Chapter 4, eating breakfast has a tremendous impact on a child's physical and academic performance as well as their behavior and attention in the classroom. Kids who eat breakfast learn better and feel better!

So why aren't young people, especially teenagers, eating breakfast? The most commonly reported reason for skipping breakfast is lack of time. Teenagers are on a schedule that literally fights with the body's natural rhythm. Their bodies want more sleep during this important period of growth and development, yet society requires them to get up at obscenely early hours and be at practice, work, or the bus stop before dawn. Given a choice between 10 more minutes of sleep or breakfast, most teens opt for the sleep. The solution is finding breakfast options that fit the schedule rather than fight the schedule. While a truly healthy breakfast has food from at least three food groups, what's most important is that kids eat something in the morning. Even if the choices aren't the most nutritious, better to have them eat something than go without breakfast at all. Table 5.1 lists a few healthy choices that kids can grab as they head out the door. See Chapter 7 for more quick breakfast ideas.

Table 5.1 Quick Breakfast Choices

Squeezable yogurts	Leftover pizza
Apples, oranges, or bananas	Orange juice
Cereal bars	Peanut butter toast
Granola bars	Bagels

Another reason teens cite for not eating breakfast, especially teenage girls, is weight control. Somewhere along the way, kids have received the mistaken notion that skipping calories at breakfast will help them control their weight. Nothing could be further from the truth. In fact, skipping breakfast or any meal usually leads to overeating at the next meal. Breakfast fuels the body's metabolism. Skipping it may result in a sluggish metabolism, making weight control more difficult.

What can parents do to get their teens eating breakfast? Parents can help by having favorite breakfast foods readily available. Ask your teenager for some ideas and involve them in the decision. Discuss with them the importance of breakfast as it relates to their personal needs. They need to know what's in it for them. Make the case for breakfast by bringing up issues that are important to teens like performance in school, performance in sports, and weight control. Stock the fridge and cabinets with healthy breakfast foods, or put breakfast bars in their coat pockets or backpacks where they'll be sure to find them. Even if it's too early in the morning for them to think about eating right when they leave the house, they may have a break before or in between classes when they can gobble a bagel.

Teens Make Healthy Meal Choices at Home and Away from Home

The nutritional status of teenagers is dependent on their ability to make healthy choices. Teens are faced with more choices today than ever before when it comes to food availability and accessibility. In addition, they have more disposable income that they can use to purchase food. Between generous allowances from parents and after-school jobs, many teens appear to have plenty of money to spend on food away from home.

At Home

At home, parents can strongly influence their kids' choices by stocking the kitchen with healthy foods that kids genuinely like. Keep the fruit bowl full, keep veggies cut up and very visible in the refrigerator. Have whole grain bagels, pitas, and crackers ready to eat with peanut butter or cheese. Teach your children some quick and easy meals to make. Attempt to always have the ingredients ready and available for them. Check out Chapter 8 for some quick and easy meal ideas, including recipes that teens can make themselves.

Packing a Lunch vs. Buying School Lunch

Chances are if your child is having trouble finding time for breakfast, he or she is also struggling to pack a lunch, healthy or not. Parents can help by packing lunches for teens or suggesting they pack lunch themselves the night before. If parents do the packing, they need to involve the teens in lunch choices. Packing a healthy lunch filled with food they don't especially like increases the chances that the lunch will end up in the garbage can at school.

Buying lunch at school is a convenient option for busy families. As we said in Chapter 4, the School Lunch Program's goal is to ensure that schools offer lunches which meet specific nutrition requirements. Teens, however, are especially susceptible to the a la carte options, like chips, fries, cookies, and sweetened beverages. A lunch made up of these items is usually low in vitamins, minerals, and fiber while high in calories and fat. Teens may not be aware of this. If families opt for the school lunch option, parents need to find out if their child is purchasing the featured meal on the menu or spending their lunch money on a la carte foods.

Eating Away from Home

When kids are away from home, they are influenced about food by many outside factors. We discussed the pros and cons of fast food in Chapters 3 and 4 and included strategies for making healthier choices for your family in a fast-food restaurant. However unlike younger children, teens are making their *own* choices at these restaurants. The parents' role is not to order for them but to help them make more informed decisions whether they are with their families or not.

Often teenagers frequent fast-food places for the social aspect more than for the food. Munching on fries and soda or coffee and muffins with a group of friends can be great fun! However, eating fast food on a regular basis can definitely lead to eating more calories and fat than teens need. In addition, they are often eating these foods in lieu of more nutritious fruits and vegetables, resulting in a pretty poor diet overall. It's unlikely that a teenager is going to stop frequenting fast-food restaurants because their parents don't like it. However with a little education and intervention on your part, they may be willing to take a closer look at the menu and make healthier decisions. An overweight teen may need your help balancing the social part of eating out with their nutrition concerns. Here are a few pointers you may want to pass on to your teen (See the section on fast food in Chapter 4 for more suggestions.):

- Choose bottled water or diet soda over regular soda.
- Share an order of fries with a friend.
- Don't super-size or if you do, share the super-size with a friend.
- Order a salad or yogurt for your meal.

Another common teen hang-out these days is the coffee or donut shop. In fact, the two fastest growing franchises this year were donut shops! While a cup of coffee and a muffin sound pretty good, the choices available these days can turn "a cup of coffee and a muffin" into a whole meal in terms of calories. Keep in mind though that it is often not a whole meal in terms of nutrition.

In these venues, calories can really start to add up without the snacker even realizing it. A seemingly innocent bran muffin can pack the same calories and grams of fat as a double cheeseburger! Even the "reduced-fat" choices often have similar numbers of calories as the regular version because of all the added sugar. For example, at a popular donut shop, the regular blueberry muffin has 490 calories. The reduced-fat blueberry muffin has 450 calories. That's not really a substantial savings on calories. A better choice is a bagel, especially a whole wheat bagel! See Table 5.2 for more details on the calories in some popular café items.

Table 5.2 Comparing Coffee Shop Choices

Item	Serving Size	Calories	Calories from Fat	Food Guide Pyramid Contribution
Cinnamon bun	1 large (Cinnabon)	750	216	Mostly fats, oils, and sweets
Cream-filled donut	1 donut	240	80	Mostly fats, oils, and sweets
Raisin bran muffin	1 large (Dunkin Donut)	490	140	Grains, including whole Grains: 2 servings
Blueberry muffin, low-fat	1 medium (Dunkin Donut)	450	120	Grains: 2 servings Fats, oils, and sweets (due to added sugar)
Wheat bagel	1 large (Dunkin Donut)	350	40	Grains: 2 servings plus 4 grams of fiber
Bagel with cream cheese	Large bagel with 2 tablespoons cream cheese	580	210	Grains: 2 servings Milk group: 1/2 serving

To increase consumption of foods from the various food groups, suggest that your teen order some 100% fruit juice or fat-free milk. Have an egg on that bagel instead of cream cheese to get a little more protein. As for the coffee, make sure your teens know what they are getting when they order hot beverages. While coffee and tea alone don't have any calories, they do have caffeine. Caffeine can act as a diuretic, making the body lose water. Also once people start adding things to coffee, like cream and sugar, they often end up with many excess calories. Watch out for specialty coffee drinks! Teens are becoming coffee drinkers and the specialty lattes and cappuccinos pack a big calorie punch. Recommend that they order these specialty drinks only occasionally and ask for low-fat or nonfat (skim) milk. See Table 5.3 for more details on coffee drinks and calories.

Table 5.3 Coffee Drinks and Calories

Black coffee	0 calories
Coffee w/2 tsp. sugar	+30 calories
Coffee w/2 T. whole milk	+20 calories
Coffee w/2 T. cream	+40 calories
Latte 12 oz.	+160 calories
Flavored coffee cappuccino 10 oz.	+230 calories

Parents Emphasize the Importance of Family Mealtime

As the kids get older, it gets much more difficult to gather everyone at the dinner table at the same time. Extracurricular activities and part-time jobs begin to disrupt mealtime, making it seem virtually impossible. Nonetheless, it is still vital that families make the effort to carve out time to eat together as a family. The reality may be that family dinners occur as infrequently as once a week, but that is still better than never!

Do you remember some of the benefits of shared meals that we discussed earlier in the book?

- Better communication
- Stronger family bonds
- Shared learning
- Improved nutrition at reduced costs

It may seem impossible to get the family together to eat now that they are teenagers, but where there is a will, there is a way. Make family mealtime a priority. That means consulting the family about their schedules and actually putting a family meal on the calendar. Be creative and flexible about when and where you eat. You may be picnicking at the ball field before a game! Involve family members in mealtime decisions. Keep meals simple and easy. This will increase the likelihood that the meal actually happens. Trying to plan an elaborate dinner may complicate things so much that you give up. Chapters 7 and 8 have some great menu-planning ideas with simple recipes for busy families. Give some of them a try.

Teens Make Healthy Snack Choices

Healthy growing teens aren't likely to go between meals without getting hungry for a snack. As we discussed in Chapter 4, snacking is actually quite beneficial as long as the snacking choices are healthy ones. However when the choices are routinely high in calories and fat, the snacks may contribute to weight issues. Teens are often making or buying snacks themselves. Parents need to step in and offer guidance to teens on what to make and what to buy, emphasizing healthy foods that the teens enjoy eating.

Planning is the key to healthy snack choices. Parents need to involve the teens in snack purchases and keep healthy snacks visible and readily available. When hungry kids come in after school or practice and it's not quite dinnertime, they are going to start foraging for snacks. Keep the fresh fruit, cut-up veggies, non-fat yogurt, and other healthy ingredients on-hand. Take a little time on the weekend to prepare a few healthy snacks with your kids, such as smoothies, granola, or pizza. Then they will be able to prepare these items themselves during your busy week.

Planning is also important if snacking is taking place outside of the home. Busy teens with after-school activities or part-time jobs will be hungry after school. They need some speedy choices available to them that are nutritious so they can avoid the vending machines and convenience stores. The Centers for Disease Control, School Health Policies and Programs Study 2000 found that nearly all (95%) high schools have vending machines. And 98% of high schools have a school store, a canteen, a snack bar, a vending machine, or a combination of these.[4] This makes it very easy for students to spend their money on less nutritious choices.

Again, the parents' role is critical. If teens do not have time to pack themselves a healthy snack, parents can help by having these items available and leaving them by their backpacks as they head out the door. If it's really impossible to provide the snacks from home, then parents need to investigate the vending machine offerings at their child's school. If the choices are all low in nutritional value (i.e., chips, cookies, and sweetened beverages), you may need to make some noise at that school about putting other items in the machines. This may seem daunting at first, but there are probably other parents who feel as you do and would be willing to jump on the band wagon and support your efforts.

Table 5.4 offers some quick snack ideas for backpacks. What's key about these snacks is that they don't need refrigeration! See Chapter 7 for more snack ideas and recipes.

Table 5.4 Backpack Snacks

Granola bars	Low fat chips
Breakfast bars	Peanut butter crackers
Mini-cereal boxes	Mini carrots
Trail mix	Apples
Pretzels	Oranges

Teens Choose Healthy Beverages

One of the highest single contributors to the typical teenager's total calorie and sugar intake is sweetened beverages. Manufacturers of soft drinks and sport drinks are cashing in on the beverage mania among today's youth. Marketing is directed at youth; product availability and choices are seemingly endless. Public schools are even reaping the economic benefits with some soft drink companies owning "pouring rights" at schools. When these relationships with corporations exist, schools get irresistible large financial rewards from the soft drink companies while the kids guzzle down hundreds of excess calories and sugar. Eighty-three percent of teenage boys and 78% of teenage girls drink soda every day![5] On average, adolescents are getting 11% of their total daily calories from soda.[6]

The solution to this growing problem is not an easy one, but parents need to attempt to guide their teens to an informed choice. Overweight teens may not realize how many extra calories they are consuming in the form of sweetened beverages. Eliminating just one 20-ounce regular soda saves the equivalent of 242 calories each day. Assuming those calories aren't replaced by something else, this change alone could result in a weight loss of up to 25 pounds in a year!

At home, parents can keep the fridge stocked with cold water or bottled water, low-calorie flavored waters, milk, and 100% juice. Offer convenient water bottles for sports and other activities. Water is still the best thirst quencher and it is best at hydrating the body. The caffeine and sugar in many sodas actually contribute to dehydration in the long run. Sports drinks are fine for teens who engage in heavy exercise lasting more than 60 minutes. Otherwise, water consumption should be encouraged.

On their own, teens must make a choice among all of these beverages. The best a parent can do is model the behavior at home (i.e., drink water instead of soda and limit sweetened beverage consumption in the house) and encourage and educate teens about better choices for beverages. Teens are going to make the decisions, a parent's job is to make sure they are making informed ones.

At the same time that teenagers are drinking more sweetened beverages, they are drinking less and less milk. In fact, only 19% of teenaged girls meet their recommended daily calcium needs.[7] This is primarily the result of decreased consumption of milk and dairy products. Bones are still growing during the teen years. It is critical that teens get the calcium they need and low-fat and fat-free dairy products can be part of a nutritious diet. Encourage teens to have a glass of non-fat milk with meals whenever possible (and do so yourself as well). Offer to teach them to prepare smoothies made with non-fat milk or yogurt. If they eat school lunch, encourage them to drink the milk that accompanies it.

Teens Don't Skip Meals

Meal-skipping is a particularly common phenomenon among teenagers. The meal most often skipped is breakfast, although teens are known to skip lunch as well. Usually the reasons cited for meal-skipping include lack of time or attempted weight control. We addressed these issues earlier in this chapter when we discussed the importance of eating breakfast. Nonetheless, some of the discussion bears repeating here.

Skipping meals will definitely not help control weight. In fact, most people who skip meals end up overeating at the next meal. "Oh, I didn't eat any breakfast, I deserve to eat this now . . ." In addition, skipping meals can confuse the metabolism so that the body starts to burn fewer calories in an effort to conserve energy. The best way to control weight is to eat healthy meals regularly and often, while getting regular exercise.

If teens are participating in vigorous exercise like track, soccer, or basketball, skipping meals will affect their performance. They need to fuel their muscles adequately to make it through practices and games. Skipping meals leaves them weaker, more fatigued, and depletes their muscles of energy stores.

Overweight Teens Are Encouraged to Make Healthy Decisions about Diets

We've intentionally avoided the concept of having children "go on a diet" in this book, favoring instead a focus on improving the nutritional quality of meals, increasing physical activity, and emphasizing family-centered behavior change. However, the emotional and social costs of being an overweight teen often lead to a desire to "diet." Parents need to be supportive of their overweight teen's efforts to control weight and offer guidance in choosing a healthy diet.

While growing teens shouldn't necessarily be restricting calories, those with a BMI above the healthy weight range may need to look at their intake more closely. Perhaps they are consuming more calories than necessary. Americans tend to eat very large portions of food. Advertisements are everywhere for mega-sizes, extra-large, and grande servings! Did you know that it takes 20 minutes for the brain to tell the stomach that it's full? In that time, people can overeat before they realize that they're not even hungry anymore. Maybe a simple hamburger will do instead of the double cheeseburger. Maybe a small order of fries is enough. While severely restricting calories is inappropriate for teens, awareness of the nutritional values (including calories) of foods may help them make better choices about how much and what they eat.

Beware of Fad Diets

Fad diets abound in our society. Visit any local or on-line bookstore and the "dieting" section is likely to be sizable. Needless to say, if any of the thousands of diets truly guaranteed healthy permanent weight loss, our national obesity epidemic would be a thing of the past. Encouraging or supporting your teen's efforts at fad diets sends the message that dieting is necessary and acceptable. A better message to send is one that involves changing and improving the nutrition and physical activity habits of the entire family.

If your teenager is starting to change his or her eating habits to lose weight, you can help by talking with them about the program they have chosen. Few, if any, weight-loss programs are appropriate for growing teens. They need sufficient calories and nutrients to maintain growth at this time. Before beginning a weight-loss program, bring your child to your physician for an assessment. During early adolescence a normal transient fatness develops in both boys and girls. This often is due to an upcoming growth spurt or, in girls, preparation for menstruation. The health care provider can determine if weight loss is truly necessary.

Any weight-loss program for teens should be undertaken with professional guidance. There are registered dietitians who are trained to assist families with weight management. A health professional will be sure to include healthy food for growth and development and emphasize an increase in physical activity. Teens and adults often are anxious to lose weight quickly and find a quick fix. Fad diets are just what they sound like. They're temporary, in and out of fashion, and don't offer a permanent solution. In some cases, fad diets can be truly dangerous to the health. How can you tell if a diet is a fad? Ask the following questions when evaluating the latest craze in weight control:

1. Does it sound too good to be true? It probably is!
2. Does it promote weight loss of more than 1–2 pounds per week? Losing more than 2 pounds per week is usually associated with water and muscle loss, not fat loss.
3. Does it say you don't need any exercise? Forget it! Any good weight control program must include exercise to maintain muscle mass and improve fitness.
4. Do you have to buy special food, pills, powders, or other products? You do? Who do you think stands to benefit the most? In the long run, it is the people selling the stuff who really benefit!

Teens are just as susceptible to the promises of miracle diets as adults are—perhaps even more so. Be sure to talk to your teen about the dangers and disappointments associated with promises of quick weight loss. We discuss fad diets in more detail in Chapter 6.

Regular Physical Activity Is Encouraged

Regular physical activity is vital for kids (and adults) of all ages. Teens, especially, will benefit from the resulting increased energy, improved academic scores, and improved self-esteem. Regular physical activity increases muscle mass, which, in turn increases metabolism. Teens need to reach the recommended goal of at least 60 minutes of physical activity per day.

Most teens who participate in team sports get the recommended 60 minutes per day of physical activity. Unfortunately, only a select group of kids go out for and are chosen to play on their school sport teams. Once kids enter middle and high school, it is more difficult to make the teams and to participate regularly in sports. In addition, at most schools physical education classes don't meet on a daily basis. Worse, some schools don't even offer physical education or offer it for only part of the year. And recess is out of the picture for this age group as well. Consequently, kids are becoming quite sedentary. In fact, children ages 8–18 spend an average of five hours per day viewing media such as television, computers, video games and videotapes.[8] When they are 12–13 years old, 69% of children participate in regular vigorous physical activity. By the time they are 18–21, the percentage drops to just 38%.[9]

For overweight teens, regular exercise can be a problem. They may suffer from embarrassment because they cannot keep up with their peers physically. Consequently, they often come up with many excuses to avoid physical activity. Parents must work with their teens to improve this situation. Teens should be encouraged to start slowly and learn to feel comfortable with their bodies. Suggest some noncompetitive activities to do together as a family. Simple walks around the neighborhood in the evening are a great way to get them moving and to spend quality time with your children. If kids are resistant or embarrassed to be seen in the neighborhood, find a more distant track or biking/hiking trail to explore as a family.

Once kids get a little stronger and more comfortable with their bodies, suggest more vigorous activities to try, such as swimming, jogging, or tennis. Offer to take a class with them to learn a new skill like dance, yoga, or spinning. Consider buying everyone in the family a pedometer. Inexpensive ones can be found at most sporting goods stores. There are many programs associated with pedometers. For example you can set a family goal of 10,000 steps per day. Teens will love the technology and fun of using the pedometer and be surprised at how much or how little exercise they are really getting.

When teens begin to feel comfortable and more self-confident about being physical, encourage them to invite a friend along and begin using the buddy system. When their friends are involved, exercise is easier and more fun. Neighborhood or backyard sports such as touch football, volleyball, kickball, baseball, or street hockey are great fun and terrific exercise. Teens can choose from a wide variety of fun and non-competitive sports such as mountain biking, rollerblading, skateboarding, skiing, or golf.

Even teens who may already be in fairly good physical condition could benefit from increased activity. This is especially true during the "off-season" for teens who play a particular sport. During this time they may find themselves becoming more sedentary and gradually getting out of shape. To boost their activity, you can suggest that they start a backyard kickball or football team, join a gym, or start a running group with friends.

Be sure to support your kids in any way you can, whether it means investing in new sneakers, or driving them to a local park or trail. Stay involved and supportive while joining in the exercise yourself. Make physical activity part of family gatherings. Start a touch football or softball game at your next picnic or holiday gathering. As always, parents must model the behavior.

A Healthy Body Image Is Encouraged and Supported

The world would be a boring place if everyone had blonde hair and blue eyes. It would be just as boring if everyone was a size four. Fortunately that is not the case and in the real world, there are many different body types. Unfortunately, the media paints a different picture. Teenagers reading magazines and watching television are exposed to an unrealistic and limited picture of what a healthy body is. They are bombarded with super-slim models and celebrities who bare their toned abs at every opportunity.

Everyone's body type is slightly different, due, in part, to his or her genetic make-up. It's what we do with that body type that matters. Everyone may not be destined to wear a size four, but everyone *can* be fit and healthy. That is truly all that matters. Parents need to guide their teens to focus on maintaining a strong, healthy and fit body that is well-nourished, not on a particular number on the scale. Teens will undoubtedly find it easier to accept themselves if their parents accept them.

Be sure to pay close attention to your teen's body image. Most eating disorders begin with a simple dieting attempt. Eating disorders are diets gone very wrong. They are extremely dangerous and must be dealt with as soon as possible. If you suspect your child has an eating disorder, seek professional help immediately. Your pediatrician should be able to refer you to the appropriate professional. See Chapter 6 for more information on eating disorders.

Parents Support the Nutrition and Physical Activity Decisions Their Teenagers Make

We've spent a great deal of time in this chapter discussing the importance of parental support of teenagers.

Teenagers are exercising their independence at every opportunity. Parents need to choose their battles carefully. Sometimes the more we, as parents, push an issue, the more the teens rebel just to spite us! This can certainly be true when it comes to what teenagers eat and how they spend their leisure time.

The teenage years are a time of experimentation and learning. Teens may suddenly want to try eating vegetarian for various religious, environmental, or nutritional reasons. They may want to embark on a stringent fitness program and be interested in the latest sports nutrition information to improve their performance. Whatever their current interest, try to be supportive. Use the information from this chapter to guide them to informed and healthy decisions. Don't worry too much about some of their choices. They may change their minds tomorrow!

So what to do about Martin?

After reading this chapter, you can see that there are many places to break the chain of events after school that may be contributing to Martin's unhealthy eating behaviors. For example, Martin is coming home from school extremely hungry. Perhaps his choices at breakfast and lunch need to be examined. He may need a more substantial and nutritious lunch to keep him from being so hungry when he gets home. But regardless of what they are eating at lunch, most teenaged boys are going to be hungry after school, so the snacks need to be ready and waiting. Martin's parents may want to re-consider the choices available to him after school. Individual servings of chips would control the portion sizes for Martin. Having cold bottled water, non-fat milk, unsweetened iced tea, or some other low calorie beverage readily available in the refrigerator could help to cut down on his sweetened beverage intake. In addition, Martin needs some limits set on TV time after school. Suggest that Martin call some buddies and start a game of pick-up basketball instead of playing video games. Finally, his parents can offer him fresh cut-up veggies or fruit to tide him over while waiting for dinner rather than cheese and crackers. Remember that even though they are teens making their own decisions, you are still the primary caregivers who are doing the grocery shopping and stocking that refrigerator. Parents still have control while the kids are eating at home!

Sources:

1. Ogden, C., Flegal, K., Carroll, M., & Johnson, C. (2000). Prevalence and trends in overweight among US children and adolescents. *The Journal of the American Medical Association*, 288, 1728–1732.
2. Samour, P.Q., Helm, K.K., & Lang, C.E. (1999). *Handbook of pediatric nutrition* (2nd ed.). New York: Aspen Publishers.
3. United States Department of Agriculture. (1994–1996). *Continuing survey of food intake by individuals* (CSFII 1994–1996). Retrieved August 26, 2003 from http://www.barc.usda.gov/bhnrc/foodsurvey/Products9496.html#individualsur-veyyears.
4. The Centers for Disease Control. (2001). School health policies and programs study 2000. *Journal of School Health,* 71, Number 7.
5. United States Department of Agriculture, Food and Nutrition Service. (January 2001). *Executive summary: Changes in children's diets, 1989–91 to 1994–1996.* Report No. CN-01-CD1.
6. See note 3.
7. Centers For Disease Control, National Center for Health Statistics. (1996). *Third national health and nutrition examination survey (NHANES III),* October 1996. Retrieved August 26, 2003 from http://www.cdc.gov/nchs/about/major/nhanes/datalink.htm#NHANESIII .
8. Kaiser Family Foundation. (1999). *Kids and media at the new millennium: A Kaiser Family Foundation report.* Retrieved August 26, 2003 from http://www.kff.org/topics.cgi.
9. Kann, L., Kinchen, S.A., Williams, B.I., Ross, J.G., Lowry, R., Grunbaum, J.A., & Kolbe L.J. (2000). Youth risk behavior surveillance—United States. *Morbidity and Mortality Weekly Report,* 49(SS-5),1–96.

CHAPTER 6

Frequently Asked Questions

What's on Your Mind?

So far in this book, we've discussed how to improve children's nutrition and physical activity habits as these habits apply to various age groups. Chapter 6 is devoted to answering the common questions we often hear from parents relating to issues of nutrition, physical activity, and overweight in children.

Top Ten Questions from Parents

1. Doesn't the Food Guide Pyramid encourage overeating? After all, isn't 6–11 servings of bread per day too many?
2. How can I really change my kid's eating choices without him noticing the decrease in calories or "putting him on a diet"?
3. My teenager says she is a vegetarian, but I am not sure this is so healthy. What should I do?
4. I'm worried that my daughter is too obsessed with what she eats and her weight. How can I tell if she has an eating disorder?

5. I keep hearing about people losing lots of weight on high-protein diets but it used to be all the talk was about eating a low-fat and high-carbohydrate diet. I'm getting confused! Which is right?
6. I know my child needs to get outside and exercise, but I don't think it is safe for my kids to go out and play without supervision and I'm usually working or busy and can't always be out there. What can I do?
7. My kids like to drink a lot of those popular new fruit teas and juice drinks. Are they good for them? Are they at least better than soda?
8. All of these "reduced-fat" and "lite" foods are pretty expensive. Is it really necessary to buy these things to improve my family's health?
9. I know we should eat together as a family, but my kids are always fighting and annoying each other at the table! It's driving me crazy!
10. It seems wherever we go, there are unhealthy snacks readily available (the movies, ball games, parties, the checkout line at the grocery store, even at the park when the ice cream man shows up!). My kids see all of this stuff and beg me to buy it. How can I say "no" all the time?

Q. Doesn't the Food Guide Pyramid Encourage Overeating? After All, Isn't 6–11 Servings of Bread Per Day Too Many?

While there are many reasons for the increased incidence of obesity in the United States, one of the primary contributors is increased portion size. Americans have lost sight of what an appropriate serving of food really is. Part of this problem began with the introduction of super-sizes and all-you-can-eat buffets at restaurants. These days, Americans expect and demand more food for their money, unaware that the individual portions of food they are being served are enough to feed entire families instead of just one person! It's hard to settle for a small popcorn at the movies, when for just 50 cents more, you can get the jumbo bucket! For many folks, their weight control issues may have less to do with *what* they are eating, than *how much* they are eating.

For example, the serving size for a bagel as defined by the USDA's Food Guide Pyramid is one ounce. Most deli-style and donut shop bagels weigh in at about four ounces. That means if you eat a bagel from a deli, you are actually eating four servings of bread! The same is true for pasta. The pyramid defines one serving as about one half-cup of cooked pasta. Most of us eat at least one cup for a portion at home so we're getting two servings. And most restaurants readily toss two cups of pasta on your plate. If you clean your plate, you're eating a hefty four servings! Yet another example of something we eat over-sized portions of is meat. The USDA defines a serving of cooked meat as about two-three ounces (a portion should be about the size of a deck of playing cards). Most Americans regularly eat three-four ounce portions (e.g., one half chicken breast is often at least three ounces and most hamburgers are at least four ounces). A typical restaurant portion of steak is at least eight ounces, if not more! So if you polish off that restaurant steak, you've just consumed four servings of meat at one meal. That's more than enough meat for the whole day!

Finally, sweetened beverages are an example of something that is often served in huge portions to children as well as adults. Years ago, sodas were sold in six- or eight-ounce bottles. Today, the average serving size is a whopping 20 ounces, with some convenience stores offering servings of 44 ounces!

As you know from reading the rest of this book, we are not saying that you should be avoiding these foods completely or never eating out. Rather, the solution lies in becoming more aware of appropriate serving sizes as well as becoming more aware of your own satiety (i.e., your sense of knowing when you are full). And you can become accustomed to taking home leftovers or splitting meals in situations where you and your family are served excessive amounts.

Why Do We Eat So Much and How Can We Stop It?

Believe it or not, young children are naturally quite good at eating appropriate portions for their age and adjusting for satiety. A recent study by USDA's Children's Nutrition Research Center at Baylor College of Medicine tested how much children aged 3–5 would eat when served different portion sizes.[1] When allowed to serve themselves, kids ate 25% less food than they ate when served large portions by an adult. And when the kids were served large portions, they ate 25% more than they ate when served normal size portions. This study suggests that the more food on a plate, the more food kids will attempt to eat. Allowing children to serve themselves portions of healthy foods appears to decrease the chances that they will overeat.

Unfortunately as kids get older, they become less sensitive to their own sense of satiety and more susceptible to portion overload. That's when they become less able to regulate their intake. This is the time for families to take control! A good place to begin is, of course, at home. For starters, parents need to become visually familiar with serving sizes. Ask yourself these questions:

- What does a half-cup of cooked pasta look like on a typical plate?
- What does one ounce of cereal look like in a standard cereal bowl?
- What does three ounces of meat look like on a dinner plate?
- How much is six ounces of fruit juice?
- How much is one tablespoon of peanut butter?

If you are not sure of the answer to any of these questions, then you may want to make it a point to measure your food for a few days. Invest in an inexpensive food scale to measure out recommended servings of meat, cheese, and other items that are measured by weight. Get out your standard measuring cups and spoons and measure the recommended servings of foods such as cereal, pasta, rice, milk, juice, or jam. Go ahead and measure out a half-cup of cooked pasta and put it on the dinner plate. Later, visualize that amount when you serve your family. A good resource to check out is USDA's "How Much are You Eating?" This guide can be downloaded from the publications and reports on the USDA Web site at www.usda.gov/cnpp. Table 6.1 offers additional practical tips for controlling portion sizes.

Table 6.1 Controlling Portion Sizes at Home and in Restaurants

At Home:

Periodically (i.e., once or twice a month) measure the typical portion you serve of the foods that you eat often. Use standard measuring cups to familiarize yourself with portion sizes and get in the habit of recognizing appropriate serving sizes.

If possible, allow family members, especially young children, to serve themselves at meals from family-style serving dishes rather than portioning amounts out for them.

When offering less nutritious items such as candy, chips, and sweetened beverages, it is a good idea to limit portion sizes:

- Measure out a serving and serve only that amount. For example, give a child two cookies instead of letting them eat an endless number out of the bag.
- Pour an eight-ounce glass of soda instead of putting the liter bottle on the table.
- Pre-portion chips and crackers into appropriate serving sizes and serve in bowls.

When Eating Out:

Avoid super-sizing.

Share your entree with another family member if the portion size is very large.

Consider ordering an appetizer instead of an entrée.

Ask for salad dressing on the side.

Order something from the menu instead of grazing at the all-you-can-eat buffet.

Have your server remove the bread basket or complimentary chips from the table instead of refilling them.

Resist the need to clean your plate; take any extra food home in a doggy bag.

Q. How Can I Really Change My Kid's Eating Choices without Him Noticing the Decrease in Calories or "Putting Him on a Diet"?

Diets are inappropriate for growing children but allowing a child to overeat and consume unreasonable portions of unhealthy foods is also inappropriate and can lead to overweight. Your child may not need to go on a restricted calorie "diet," but their food intake could perhaps benefit from an overhaul. Let's take a look at a sample day's intake for a 10-year-old child and see how making a few minor changes can bring the calorie intake into a more appropriate range for his age and activity level.

An average recommended caloric intake for a lightly active 10-year-old is around 2500 calories per day. See Table 6.2 for a comparison of appropriate and inappropriate daily menus for a child of this age. You can see that with a few simple substitutions and portion changes, the calorie intake can easily be reduced to within normal limits and the nutrition can be improved. No child eating the modified diet would feel the least bit deprived or feel that he or she was being placed on a "diet."

Table 6.2 Daily Food Makeover for a 10-Year-Old

Original Diet	Modified Diet
BREAKFAST	**BREAKFAST**
Cap'n Crunch® cereal, 2 cups	Cheerios® cereal, 2 cups
Whole milk, 1 cup	Low-fat milk, 1 cup
Orange juice, 8 ounces	Orange juice, 8 ounces
SNACK	**SNACK**
Cheese puffs, 2 ounces	Pretzels, 1 ounce
Juice drink, 1 pouch	Mini carrots, 8
LUNCH	**LUNCH**
Ham and cheese sandwich on white bread	Ham and cheese sandwich on whole wheat bread,
Potato chips, 2 ounces	Potato chips, 1 ounce
Chocolate sandwich cookies, 3	Apple, fresh, 1 medium
Whole milk, 8 ounces	low-fat chocolate milk, 1 cup
Applesauce cup, 1	Chocolate sandwich cookies, 2
SNACK	**SNACK**
Sports drink, 20 ounces	Banana smoothie (see recipe in Chapter 8), 1
Fruit roll-up, 1	Cereal bar, 1

Table 6.2 Daily Food Makeover for a 10-Year-Old *(Continued)*

Original Diet	Modified Diet
DINNER	**DINNER**
Fast-food cheeseburger, 1	Fast-food cheeseburger
Fast-food fries, 1 large	Fast-food fries, 1/2 large
Soda, 16 ounces	low-fat milk, 1 cup
SNACK/DESSERT	**SNACK**
Chocolate ice cream, 1 cup	Fudgesicle® frozen bar, 1
TOTALS	**TOTALS**
3150 calories, 35% of calories from fat, 60% of dietary fiber recommendation	2470 calories, 26% of calories from fat, 100% of dietary fiber recommendation

Q. My Teenager Says She Is a Vegetarian, but I Am Not Sure This Is So Healthy? What Should I Do?

Vegetarian diets are becoming increasingly popular for a variety of reasons including taste, ethics, religion, and health. Vegetarian diets, when followed correctly, are usually healthy diets, high in fiber, fruits, vegetables, and whole grains. As a result, vegetarians tend to be leaner than non-vegetarians and have lower incidences of heart disease and certain types of cancer. This is only true, however, if they are following a healthy vegetarian diet. Just as there are poor choices in a non-vegetarian diet, there can be poor choices in a vegetarian diet. If you consider yourself a vegetarian, but fill your diet with "junk food", then vegetarianism is not going to make you any healthier. If you are a vegetarian or are considering vegetarianism for your family, you can learn how to choose a healthy vegetarian diet.

A typical vegetarian does not eat meat, fish, and poultry. Vegans are vegetarians who abstain from eating or using all animal products, including milk, cheese, other dairy items, eggs, wool, silk, and leather. A well-planned vegetarian diet can meet all known nutrient needs if followed consistently and conscientiously. The key to a healthy vegetarian diet, as with any other diet, is to eat a wide variety of foods, including fruits, vegetables, plenty of leafy greens, whole grain products, nuts, seeds, and legumes. As with all diets, if you are a vegetarian, you should limit your intake of sweets and high-fat foods, especially foods with trans fatty acids. Finally, everyone must include regular physical activity in your lifestyle. There is a vegetarian food guide pyramid (Figure 6.1) to assist vegetarians in planning a healthy diet.

Children and Vegetarianism

A vegetarian diet can be appropriate for children if it is well-planned. It is important to include enough calories and protein to support growth. In addition, certain nutrients tend to be lower or lacking in a vegetarian diet and must be taken into consideration when planning a vegetarian diet. These include iron, calcium, vitamin B_{12}, vitamin D, and zinc.

Protein

Vegetable protein usually does not have all of the essential amino acids so it is referred to as an incomplete protein. However, often if one vegetable or grain may be missing an amino acid, another vegetarian food may have it. If a vegetarian eats them together, he or she can get all the essential amino acids. This is called complimenting proteins. When you compliment proteins, you combine proteins from different vegetarian sources so that all of the essential amino acids are available. Vegetarians do not have to combine these items at the same meal, but they do need to be aware over the course of a day that they have eaten an appropriate combination of food items. In this way, eating a variety of plant-based foods can provide vegetarians with all the essential amino acids.

If the vegetarians in your home are not vegans and they eat eggs and/or milk, they don't need to worry about

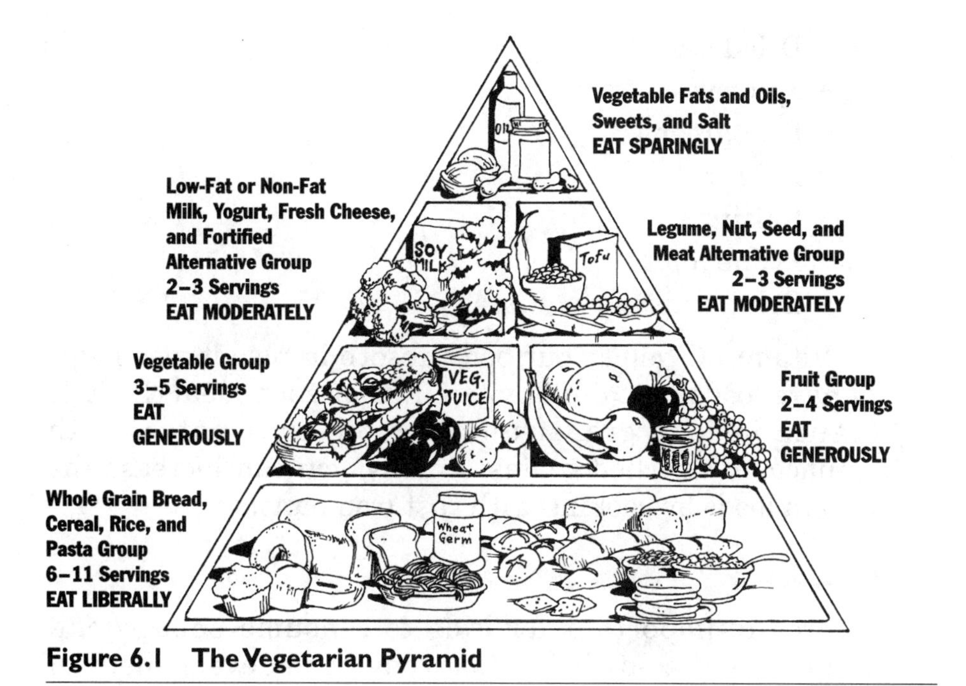

Figure 6.1 The Vegetarian Pyramid

complimenting proteins because eggs, milk, yogurt, cheese, etc. are great complete protein sources. Here are some common vegetarian food combinations. Each represents a complete protein:

- Rice and beans
- Corn tortillas and black beans
- Peanut butter on whole grain bread

Iron

Plant foods do contain iron. However the iron in plants is not as well absorbed by your body as the iron in meat, poultry, and fish. Consequently, vegetarians need to eat a little more iron than non-vegetarians. Many breads and cereals are *enriched* with iron so including enriched grains in your vegetarian diet helps to increase iron intake. Other plant sources of iron include:

- Dried beans
- Spinach
- Beet greens
- Bulgur
- Raisins
- Prune juice
- Dried fruit

Vitamin C helps your body absorb iron so it also helps to have foods containing vitamin C at each meal. Include orange juice, a grapefruit, broccoli, or tomatoes with spinach or enriched grains. Finally, you can increase the iron in foods by cooking with cast iron pans!

Calcium

It's really important for kids to consume enough calcium since it contributes to strong bone development. A vegetarian who eats dairy products probably is getting enough calcium from drinking milk, and eating yogurt, ice cream, and other foods high in calcium. Vegans need to actively seek out high-calcium vegan foods. A vegan's intake of calcium is likely to be low unless he or she consciously works to consume high-calcium foods. Everyone, vegetarians and non-vegetarians alike, should try to include at least three sources of calcium in their diet each day. A few plant sources of calcium include:

- Leafy green vegetables, such as collard greens, turnip greens, kale
- Broccoli
- Calcium-fortified tofu
- Calcium-fortified soy milk
- Calcium-fortified breads and waffles
- Calcium-fortified orange juice

Vitamin B_{12}

We all need vitamin B_{12} for nerve function. Although plant foods have some B_{12}, they are not a good source. It is recommended that vegetarians, and vegans in particular, take a B_{12} supplement or make sure that they eat foods that are fortified with B_{12} to help meet these requirements. There are vegetarian products, such as cereals, available that are fortified with B_{12}.

Vitamin D

Vitamin D works with calcium to keep bones strong. It's tough for everyone to get enough vitamin D in their diet unless fortified products are consumed. The one fortified product most people consume is milk. Vegans obviously need another source. If there is a vegan in your household, buy fortified soy milk or cereals.

Everyone can make vitamin D in their body if they get some sun exposure. Just 5 to 15 minutes of sun exposure a day is enough! If you spend any more time than that in the sun, be sure to wear sunscreen.

Zinc

Zinc is vital to growth and development. The best source of zinc is red meat. Many plant sources of zinc are not very well absorbed. Some plant sources that are acceptable are:

- Whole grains
- Legumes
- Nuts
- Tofu

If you don't think you and your family members are getting enough zinc from your diet, you should talk to your doctor about a multivitamin/mineral supplement that contains zinc.

Vegetarians Eating Out

One of the hardest things about being a vegetarian is eating out especially at fast-food restaurants or the school cafeteria. If your child is a lacto-ovo vegetarian (i.e. eats eggs and drinks milk), this won't be so difficult. Be sure to include a milk, yogurt, or cheese source in your child's meal, along with some whole grains and fruits and/or vegetables. In a school lunch, this could be yogurt, a piece of fruit, or a bagel in addition to any other vegetarian items you choose. Vegans need to do some advance planning and may need to bring lunch from home if the school can't accommodate their special needs. Ask the food service director at school if they offer vegetarian dishes.

In a restaurant, the issues are similar. A vegetarian can usually get a milk, bread, and salad at most restaurants, even fast food restaurants. They can also often find baked potatoes or rice and ask for cheese to accompany them. Meatless pizza or bean burritos can be great choices and are readily available. What a vegetarian wants to avoid is choosing less nutrient-dense foods just because they are meat-free. A soda and a large order of fries may be vegetarian but they are not the most nutritious choices!

A Family Divided

Some families may have one or more members who are vegetarians while the remaining members of the family are not. The best way to handle this is to involve *all* family members in menu planning and grocery shopping. Familiarize non-vegetarians with vegetarian choices. Have the non-vegetarians sample the vegetarian dishes. The rest of the family may actually like some of these items.

Lots of everyday dishes like pasta, pizza, tacos, and salads can be prepared to serve to both vegetarians and non-vegetarians. You can't be expected to short-order cook for your family. If everyone stays flexible, creative, and respectful of each other's wishes, vegetarianism shouldn't create a problem!

Q. I'm Worried That My Daughter Is Too Obsessed with What She Eats and Her Weight. How Can I Tell If She Has an Eating Disorder?

Eating disorders are dieting gone very wrong. Although the causes of eating disorders are quite complex and often have strong psychological roots unrelated to food, many eating disorders start with attempts at dieting. The dieter becomes obsessed or fixated on success with the diet. They begin to lose sight of a healthy weight and develop a distorted body image.

The most common eating disorders are anorexia nervosa, bulimia nervosa, and binge eating. Anorexia nervosa, often called "anorexia" is characterized by eating very small amounts of food combined with excessive exercising. Anorexics usually are extremely thin, with a body weight 15% below a defined healthy weight (based on the person's age and height). Bulimia nervosa or "bulimia" is characterized by eating or binging on excessive amounts of food followed by purging through the use of self-induced vomiting or laxative abuse. Bulimics are usually of normal weight or are slightly overweight. Binge eating is characterized by eating excessive amounts of food (i.e., an entire box of cookies in one sitting), usually in secret. Binge eaters are often overweight.

Eating disorders are most often seen in teenaged or college-aged females. However, eating disorders are now being diagnosed in children as young as 9 or 10 years of age and also in males. Regardless of the type of eating disorder or the age of the child, eating disorders are very serious and life-threatening. Anorexics can become so thin and weak that they literally starve to death. Bulimics can upset the electrolyte balance in their bodies from excessive vomiting and suffer from heart attacks. Parents need to take the situation seriously and get professional help for their child as soon as possible. It's important for parents to be able to recognize some signs of a potential eating disorder. The following table lists some signs and symptoms of eating disorders. If you are concerned, you need to confront your child and get them professional help. Your pediatrician should be able to refer you to a specialist. You will also find helpful information about eating disorders at www.anad.org.

Table 6.3 Signs and Symptoms of Eating Disorders

Common Behaviors of People with Anorexia Nervosa
Prolonging mealtimes; cutting food in very small pieces and moving it around the plate
Secretive eating
Avoiding certain foods, such as red meat, fats, desserts, and breads
Eating as little as possible during the day; saving eating for nighttime
Choosing foods that have few calories so they are therefore able to eat more (salads, low-fat yogurt, gum, sugar-free beverages)
Eating as few as 300 to 1000 calories per day
Common Behaviors of People with Bulimia Nervosa
Low fat intake
Skipping meals and irregular eating habits
Limiting food choices
Low-carbohydrate food intake when not bingeing
Considering certain foods to be "good" or "bad"
Eating secretly
Overexercising
When bingeing • Eating high-carbohydrate and high-fat foods • Bingeing in private • Binge occurs usually in late afternoon or at night • Feeling guilty when binging • Often bingeing on convenience foods (not taking the time to stop and prepare something)

Prevention of eating disorders is the goal. Parents can help by encouraging lifelong healthy eating and physical activity habits. Most importantly, parents need to emphasize a positive self-image and acceptance of different body types. Mothers especially need to be careful of obsessive dieting, as young girls tend to model their mothers' behaviors.

As we have said previously, putting children "on diets" is unhealthy and only serves to send the message that they are different and that their looks are somehow unacceptable. The message we want to send is that all body types are acceptable as long as we eat healthy and get regular exercise. The emphasis is on health and fitness, not the numbers on the bathroom scale!

Q. I Keep Hearing About People Losing Lots of Weight on High-Protein Diets, but It Used to Be All the Talk Was about Eating a Low-Fat and High-Carbohydrate Diet. I'm Getting Confused! Which Is Right?

Lots of people these days are trying the high-protein approach to weight loss, eating seemingly endless amounts of bacon, eggs, and burgers and dropping pounds. It is true that switching from a high-carbohydrate diet to a high-protein diet will result in an initial quick weight loss. Carbohydrate holds water; therefore, reducing carbohydrate intake usually results in a quick loss of water, which shows up on the scale.

However, long-term weight loss can only be achieved if calorie intake is lower than energy needs, regardless of the calorie source. You can lose weight eating ice cream all day if the total calories you consume are less than what you need to maintain your weight! But will you be healthy? While protein is a vital nutrient, most Americans get plenty of it without going on a special diet. Staying on a high-protein diet over time can be a strain on the kidneys. Also, if a high-protein diet doesn't include enough fruits, vegetables, and whole grains, many key vitamins, minerals, and fiber will be missing. Some experts have also voiced concerns about high-protein diets being high in saturated fat content. Diets high in saturated fat have been linked with increased risk of heart disease and certain cancers.

In contrast, the low-fat high-carbohydrate approach to weight loss hasn't been particularly successful either. A diet too low in fat can leave a dieter feeling hungry soon after eating. High-carbohydrate diets can be healthy if the carbohydrates are primarily whole grains, fruits, and vegetables as opposed to simple carbohydrates like white bread and pasta. A diet featuring too many simple carbohydrates can also leave the dieter feeling hungry soon after eating.

The only real way to lose weight permanently involves calorie intake control and good old-fashioned exercise. Any program, pill, or formula that promises quick weight loss with minimal effort is likely a scam. After all, if the "magic bullet" really existed, there wouldn't be the obesity problem there is.

Kids, especially, need to avoid drastic programs and dietary modifications like a high-protein diet. Their growing bodies need the balance of all the nutrients we get from a variety of foods, all eaten in moderation.

Q. I Know My Child Needs to Get Outside and Exercise, but I Don't Think It Is Safe for My Kids to Go Out and Play Without Supervision and I'm Usually Working or Busy and Can't Be Out There. What Can I Do?

You're right to be concerned about your children's safety. It is not appropriate to throw your kids out the back door to play in every neighborhood. But that doesn't mean you should give up on boosting your family's activity level. Perhaps you can schedule family fun time on the weekends and take your kids to a safe park or playground to play. To increase activity during the week when you are at work, find out about supervised games and athletic activities at your child's school. There may be after-school programs with an emphasis on physical activity. In addition, there may be inexpensive programs in your community affiliated with Boys & Girls clubs, the YMCA, and local parks & recreation programs. You may be able to coordinate with other parents to transport the kids to one of these programs. If none of these options are available to you and your children must stay inside, it still doesn't mean they need to sit in front of the television. Playing hide and seek, "dress-up," dancing, charades, and so on—all involve movement and are better (and more fun!) than sitting around!

Q. My Kids Like to Drink a Lot of Those Popular New Fruit Teas and Juice Drinks. Are They Good for Them? Are They at Least Better Than Soda?

Unless the label clearly says "100% fruit juice," the majority of juice drinks and fruit teas have little or no actual fruit juice. What they have plenty of is sugar! Consumption of sweetened beverages like these along with soda and fruit punch has risen dramatically over the past few years. A recent study conducted by researchers at Cornell University and referenced in the Journal of Pediatrics found that drinking too much soda and other sweetened beverages may cause obesity in children.[2] These findings are alarming. Researchers followed 30 children ages 6–12 for a two-month period. They found that children who drank more than 12 ounces of sweetened drinks per day gained significantly more weight over the two-month period (2.5 pounds) than the kids who drank less than 6 ounces per day. The children who drank more than 16 ounces per day also consumed less milk, protein, calcium, and vitamin A than the other children did.

The bottom line is you should serve low-fat milk with meals, occasional juice with snacks, and lots of water every day. Limit consumption of sweetened beverages and stock the fridge with the drinks you want to encourage your child to consume to be healthier and maintain a healthier weight.

Q. All of These "Reduced-Fat" and "Lite" Foods Are Pretty Expensive. Is It Really Necessary to Buy These Things to Improve My Family's Health?

The short answer to this question is "no"! Here's why…

Years ago, dietitians could safely recommend that people consume less fat in order to lose weight. After all, fat has more calories per gram than either carbohydrate or protein. The low-fat message backfired however. What happened was that the food industry responded overwhelmingly and created thousands of products that have lower fat content than regular versions. Unfortunately this did not result in a thinner society! People began eating these products in abundance thinking that low-fat meant no-calorie and their calorie consumptions actually increased. Add to this the fact that fat helps make your stomach feel full and a diet too low in fat can leave you feeling hungry which leads to even more overeating!

Fast forward to today! Our recommendations as dietitians have become more sophisticated. Everyone needs some fat in his or her diet. Some fats are better for you than others, such as monounsaturated fats like canola and olive oil. Other fats, such as saturated fats and trans fats, are potentially harmful if consumed in excess. It's not necessary to purchase reduced-fat or fat-free foods. Go ahead and buy the items you want on occasion, but pay closer attention to the portion size and calories per serving. Better to have one or two regular chocolate chip cookies than to eat ten reduced-fat chocolate chip cookies. Fill your shopping cart with lots of fruits, vegetables, whole grains, lean meats, beans, and low-fat dairy products. If your family fills up on these good-for-them foods, the rest of the items (snacks and treats!) are less necessary. And since the "treats' are also usually more expensive you'll end up saving money and eating healthier.

Q. I Know We Should Eat Together as a Family, but My Kids Are Always Fighting and Annoying Each Other at the Table! It's Driving Me Crazy!

Remember "Leave it to Beaver?" At the dinner table, June wore a dress and heels and Wally and Beaver sat politely, eating everything on their plate, and chewing with their mouths closed. Yikes!

The reality is that kids will be kids and some mealtime ruckus is to be expected in all families. However, making the mealtime as pleasant as possible helps to ensure that your family gets the most out of mealtime. The kids should sit at the table, eat slowly, chew thoroughly, and learn to recognize when they are full. In addition to modeling these positive behaviors for your kids, there are numerous nutritional benefits you're giving your kids by eating together as a family.

Of course, the logistics of gathering as a family for the evening meal require planning and consistency. The family needs to have defined rules about eating behaviors and expectations at the table. Discuss all of these issues at a time separate from the meal. Children need to know the rules in advance and have an opportunity to practice and apply them. Chewing with mouths closed, elbows off the table, saying "please" and "thank you," and using good manners are some things that kids need time to work on and improve upon as they get older. Parents need to stick to the rules and be consistent with discipline. If the rules are broken, enforce the pre-arranged punishment quickly and without discussion. With a little work, your family mealtime should quickly become a more pleasant event.

One family we know found that simply moving the dinner meal from the kitchen to the dining room alleviated a lot of the arguments between the kids. Their dining room table was bigger and the kids were further apart from each other, allowing less opportunity to touch and pester each other. If this isn't possible for your family, consider rearranging the seating to keep arguing siblings apart.

The mealtime itself is not the time to spend constantly bickering and reprimanding the kids. Focus on keeping the conversation fun and keeping all the family involved in the discussion. Take the time to enjoy the food and each other.

Q. It Seems Wherever We Go, There Are Unhealthy Snacks Readily Available (the Movies, Ball Games, Parties, the Checkout Line at the Grocery Store, Even at the Park When the Ice Cream Man Shows Up!). My Kids See All of This Stuff and Beg Me to Buy It. How Can I Say "No" All the Time?

We certainly do seem to live in a food-obsessed society, don't we? It seems that every occasion is associated with eating and food. Some of this is perfectly normal and acceptable. However, when it seems that there are "special occasions" every day, you may need to be a little more proactive as a parent.

First of all, you needn't feel compelled to say "no" all the time. In fact, you need to say "yes" periodically or your children will begin to view certain foods as completely forbidden and start to crave them even more. With that said, you do still need to decide when to say no and when to say yes. Planning ahead and involving the kids in your decision-making can prevent hassles later.

For example, when going to the movies, decide ahead of time exactly how much, if any, snacks the child will be allowed to have and tell them before you go, "I'll buy you popcorn, but not soda." Or, "You may have soda, but no candy with it." If they argue when you get there, they get nothing! Do the same thing when bringing the kids to the grocery store. Allow them to choose one item, perhaps a special cereal or snack or dessert. If they ask for a second item when you're there, ask them to choose which item they want more. For example, in the check-out line, when they ask for candy, you say, "If I buy you candy, we'll need to put back the chips you chose. Which do you want?" Avoid giving kids more than two choices. It becomes too difficult for them to choose and opens up too many issues for the parent.

Also, make sure the kids have eaten before you go to events that feature lots of snacks. They will really bug you if they are hungry. Eat lunch or dinner before the movies, have a healthy snack before going to the grocery store. Pack healthy snacks to have in the car for those stops at the park or ball games. This will help you to avoid trips to the concession stand or the ice cream truck.

It's Time to Cook

Now that you have armed yourself with lots of nutrition and physical activity information and had your questions answered (hopefully!), you are ready to tackle menu planning. The next two chapters in the book deal with basic issues of menu planning and food preparation. In order to feed your family healthy food, you need to do some planning and be prepared to make healthy shopping and cooking decisions. With a little advance preparation and know-how, you'll be ready to enjoy a new healthy and active lifestyle with your family.

Read on and enjoy!

Sources:

1. Fisher, J.O., Rolls, B.J., & Birch, L.L. (2003). Children's bite size and intake of an entrée are greater with large portions than with age-appropriate or self-selected portions. *American Journal of Clinical Nutrition,*77, 1164–70.
2. Mrdjenovic, G. & Levitsky, D.A. (2002). Nutritional and energetic consequences of sweetened drink consumption in 6-13-year old children. *Journal of Pediatrics,* 142, 604–610.

CHAPTER 7

Menu Planning

Making Time to Prepare Healthy Meals

Justin is just starting high school and is having lots of trouble getting up so early to go to school. His routine is to sleep as late as he possibly can, then roll out of bed, jump into his clothes, and run to the bus. His mom and dad are extremely concerned that he is not eating breakfast. Justin explains to them that he just doesn't have the time. What should Justin and his family do to get school days off to a better nutritional start given the reality of their busy lives?

Menu Planning Is Important for Every Family

Although it can be frustrating trying to find the time to make healthy meals for your family and satisfy everyone in the household, it is important for all family members to have three to six meals per day. We believe, as most experts do, that eating well and often (in moderation) is crucial to fueling your body throughout the day. Studies have shown that our metabolism is more efficient when we eat small frequent meals. Unfortunately, meal planning becomes even more challenging as children grow because parents have less control over what kids eat outside of the home. In this chapter, we will provide you with some healthy menu planning tips to provide nutritious meals for your family that fit into your busy lifestyle.

Top Ten Healthy Meal Planning Tips

The following list features some basic starting points to help you fit menu planning and cooking into your family's busy lives.

1. Be prepared—have "the basics" available at home.
2. Plan in advance—think through your week's activities and see what will work in your schedule.
3. Consult your family about menu choices.
4. Shop regularly.
5. Read food labels.
6. Start the day with breakfast.
7. Have a healthy lunch.
8. Eat dinner as a family.
9. Have healthy snacks readily available.
10. Make good choices when eating out or bringing home prepared foods.

Be Prepared—Have "the Basics" Available at Home

It's important to have "the basics" on hand. The number of meals Americans eat away from home has increased by 50% per person in the last 20 years. Needless to say this is not only generally a more expensive option but often a less nutritious one as well. Meals eaten away from home tend to be higher in calories. Foods that are bought already prepared or are quick-to-prepare may have hidden calories due to processing. You can improve your family's nutrition (and help family members achieve or maintain a healthy weight) by cooking at home more often. This will be a more realistic option if you take the time to plan ahead.

What Are "the Basics"?

How many times have you been running late only to find that you must stop at the grocery store to pick up something so you can make the dinner you planned? Or maybe you are one of the many people who do not even know what they will be serving for dinner when 4 p.m. rolls around. If you find yourself in either of these positions (and who doesn't occasionally?), you can improve your situation by keeping the following items on hand. By having these menu staples always available, you'll be able to easily put together a quick and nutritious meal with less last-minute shopping and lots less stress!

Produce

- Onions
- Potatoes
- Carrots
- Fruits that don't spoil easily (apples, oranges, etc.)

Protein Foods

- 1-pound packages of ground beef or turkey in separate containers (freezer)
- Boneless skinless chicken breasts, one half breast for each member of your family (freezer)
- Eggs
- Canned tuna
- Cheese, sliced
- Cheese, shredded (You can even keep this in the freezer so it will last longer.)
- Bacon
- Milk

Frozen Foods

- Variety of vegetables (Choose your family favorites!)
- Flour or corn tortillas (Yes, you can freeze them!)
- Variety of meats and cheeses (See above list.)

Non-Perishable Items

- Tomato sauce
- Jars of pasta sauce
- 1-pound boxes of pasta
- Canned soup
- Rice
- Bread
- Mayonnaise
- Salsa
- Canned fruit
- Taco chips
- Taco seasoning mix
- Instant pudding

If you have these items in your kitchen, you'll be able to put together a meal in no time at all. Tables 7.1 and 7.2 provide examples of quick dinners featuring these ingredients, that are easy to prepare and your family will enjoy.

Table 7.1 Making Meals from the Basics

Sample Dinner
Bowl of chicken noodle soup
Grilled cheese sandwich on whole wheat bread
Carrot sticks
Canned peaches
Nutritional analysis: 435 calories, 33% of calories from fat, good source of vitamins A and C and fiber

*You might think that the fat content for the above meal is somewhat high since the Dietary Guidelines recommend you get only 30% of your calories from fat. However, remember this is only one meal. Even if you eat this meal for dinner, your average fat intake for the day could easily fall within the recommendations depending on your other meals. Also when you look at nutrient analysis for your own diet you should average your nutrient intake over the course of at least three days. So a dinner like this can fit into a healthy day of eating.

Table 7.2 Another Meal from the Basics

Sample Dinner
Frittata (see recipe in Chapter 8)
Tortilla chips (1 ounce)
Green beans
Apple
Nutritional analysis: 478 calories, 23% of calories from fat, good source of vitamin C and fiber

There is nothing wrong with having hamburger patties, veggie burgers, or tuna sandwiches for dinner. How about breakfast foods for dinner? The family might really enjoy bacon and eggs one night. Most teens and children love pancakes and waffles. Serve them with fruit and low-fat milk and you have a delicious and nutritious meal. If you use your imagination a little and keep these staples readily available, you'll always be prepared to make a quick meal.

Plan in Advance

Think through your week's activities and see what will work with your family's schedule. American lives have certainly changed over the past several years. There are many single-parent families and families with two working parents. Single-parent families have increased from 9.1% in 1961 to 27.3% in 1998. From 1980 to 2000, the percentage of women in the workforce increased from approximately 52% to 62%. More people than ever have very demanding jobs with long work hours and lots of stress. This translates into families not having much time for food preparation. As a result more meals are eaten away from home. In addition, people often do not have the cooking skills that previous generations had. Many people did not have cooking role models or a lifestyle that permitted them to develop cooking skills. There is nothing wrong with this. We just need to realize where we are and plan accordingly.

We also live in a world where our children are involved in more and more activities outside the home. Many children have one or more planned activities everyday—piano lessons, soccer, baseball, dance, or even all of these things! It seems that children are busier than ever and the more activities the children are involved in, the more crammed the family schedule becomes.

So who has time to plan a meal? You do. Take a few minutes, perhaps over the weekend, and think through what each member of your family has scheduled for the week. What time will everyone be home in the evenings? Be realistic! If you need to be at a game at 6 p.m. and don't arrive home until 5:30 p.m., you don't have time to make an elaborate meal. In certain cases, you may need to feed the kids a granola bar and a cup of low-fat milk to eat in the car on the way to the field and stop for a quick supper later. Certain times of the year are more hectic than others and eating out may be necessary periodically but better planning can make this type of evening the exception rather than the rule.

It is very important for you to take the time to plan meals if you want your family to eat healthy meals. Meals eaten at home tend to be more nutritious than meals eaten away from home. Decide what nights you just cannot make a meal, accept the fact that your family will eat prepared foods those nights, and plan what you will make for dinner on the other nights. If you have time to cook more on weekends, cook a meal that might take longer to prepare then and use some of the leftovers during the week. In the sample month's menu in Chapter 8, we demonstrate how you can use leftovers from the weekend in easy weekday recipes. For example, if you make a *Roasted Chicken* on Sunday, you can easily make the *Chicken and Vegetable Stir-Fry* during the week. You can also use leftover cooked chicken to make *Chicken Enchiladas.* Many stir-fry recipes adapt very well to using leftovers—try the *Beef and Broccoli Stir-Fry.* Stir-frying is a very healthy method of cooking. You add little additional fat and can quickly prepare a meal with both a source of protein and lots of yummy vegetables—what could be healthier?

Another trick we like is doubling a recipe and freezing half to use another time. The *Baked Ziti with Mini Meatballs* in Chapter 8 is a perfect recipe to double. You'll find if you make the sauce recipe you will have plenty to freeze and use later. Just make sure to freeze the sauce in containers that suit your family's needs. You'll then have homemade tomato sauce that will be available another time to toss with pasta for a quick supper. You can even turn it into a meat sauce by adding ground beef or turkey. It really is best to try to plan a week's worth of meals in advance. If you do this, you are able to plan how you can best use leftovers and figure out what kind of meal is realistic to prepare on each night. You should even plan the nights you may need to eat out or pick something up. Making restaurant or take-out meals planned events means you will be less likely to rely on them as often. Having them on the family calendar will also help your kids understand that you are not going "cold-turkey" when it comes to eating out at their favorite places. When they know they get to go out for pizza after soccer practice on Tuesday they may be more open to trying new foods at home on Monday.

Consult Your Family about Menu Choices

When we learn about team-building in the workplace, we are always taught that on a successful team everyone is informed about what is going to occur and why. Why not apply this rule of thumb to your home? Everyone likes to know what's going on, including kids! You might have a better chance of getting your children to try new foods if you get them involved. Why not ask each family member to pick out a new food item that they would like to try during the week? Depending on their age, you might even want to get your children involved in food preparation. We have found that our kids truly enjoy having input into family meal planning. It can help build self-esteem for children when they see that they can be successful at a real-world adult activity like preparing food. As an added bonus, it might actually take some of the pressure off of you!

If you want your children to eat healthy, you will want to take steps to make sure that they like the healthy foods you serve. Getting their buy-in in the planning stages can help ensure that this is the case. Overweight children especially should be included in meal planning to reinforce the concept that they are in control of what and how much they are eating. Allowing overweight children opportunities to "take charge" of their relationship with food can help them feel less powerless about their weight and the amount and kinds of foods they eat. Instead of feeling like victims who are not "allowed" certain foods, they can feel like they are sharing responsibility for their family's good health.

Don't be a short-order cook! It is much easier to plan one meal for everyone, and you can do this more readily if you get your kids input early in the planning and cooking process. Of course, we all know that some kids are fussier than others. If you plan it correctly, you can offer new foods that you enjoy even if they are unfamiliar to your child. Have your child try the new food but don't insist that they eat a prescribed amount. When you make a new entrée, serve it with side dishes that you know your child will like. A child will not starve if bread and milk are available. If your child is hungry later because they did not like a new food you served, offer a bowl of cereal or a sandwich as a bedtime snack. If your child is overweight, it is important to have healthy evening snack options available so that he or she does not just snack on junk food throughout the night after choosing not to eat a nutritious meal.

Shop Regularly

With our busy schedules it makes sense to go to the store as infrequently as possible. Without proper planning, you may find yourself spending too much of your valuable time on multiple "quick" trips to the grocery store each week. Plan ahead as discussed above and make a grocery list and you may be able to avoid the endless cycle of stopping at the store every night. Many people enjoy shopping at the wholesale clubs because they can stock up on foods they use regularly and save money. There are usually good buys on many items that fit well into our busy lives including individually packaged food items like pudding, baby carrots, fruit cups, and applesauce. While these are great places to save money, many shoppers find that they need to supplement this type of shopping because these stores may not have everything they need or the quantities are just too large for smaller families.

For many of us it makes sense to go to the grocery store weekly to supplement monthly warehouse market trips. If you have a week of menus planned you are armed to shop efficiently! If you shop with your weekly menu in hand, you will have to stop less frequently during the week and save yourself both time and money. You also will not be frantically thinking at 4 p.m. about what to make for dinner each night—and this will be less stressful for you and the whole family. For some people, shopping once a week may be too frequent and a trip every two weeks works better.

Do whatever works best for you. Just remember to plan your menus ahead and write out your shopping list accordingly. It really does work.

Read Food Labels

Since you are reading this book, you are obviously concerned about your family's health. Learning to read a food label will help you make healthy food choices for your family. Once you know how to decipher the labels, you'll find that lots of nutrition information is available on the packaging of your favorite foods.

Nutrition Facts Label

Although most people refer to this as the "food label," the real name is "Nutrition Facts Label." Since 1990, federal regulation has required food companies to display nutrition information on food items in a specific and consistent manner. We've broken down the Nutrition Facts Label and an explanation of each section follows. Obviously, there is a great deal of information on the shelf in your local grocery store. Take your time and look at food labels. Be aware that some items do not have food labels, such as fresh produce, meat, fish, and poultry. Ask the manager if you'd like to see nutrition information for these items.

Serving Size / Servings per Container

This indicates what a normal adult serving size of this food product is and how many servings are in the container. This information is key to weight control! If you eat a whole can of an item, and the label states there are two servings per container, that means you need to multiply everything by two—including the calories!

Calories

This section provides information about ONE single serving! This is where you will find how many *calories are in one serving* and how many of those *calories come from fat*. Many people today are concerned about *percent of fat* for a food item. This information is not listed specifically on the food label, so you'll need to do some math if you want this information! It's really pretty easy. All you need to do is divide the number of fat calories by the total calories. If an item has 300 total calories and 75 of them are fat calories, then 25% of the calories are from fat (75 divided by 300 is .25 or 25%).

Nutrients Important to Your Health

Fat, Carbohydrate, and Protein amounts are listed for each serving in grams. If you want to know about calories for each nutrient, you'll have to do a little more math. Just multiply the number of grams times the calories per gram below.

- Fat = 9 calories per gram
- Carbohydrate = 4 calories per gram
- Protein = 4 calories per gram

Cholesterol, Sodium, Sugars, and *Fiber* are listed because they are of great concern to people. Recommended amounts for all of these items are listed in the Dietary Guidelines 2000.

Percentage of Daily Value

The *Daily Value* (DV) tells you how a serving of the food contributes to your daily intake of various nutrients. It is based on a "reference intake" of *2,000 calories per day.* For example, if a label states that a food has a DV for carbohydrate of 10%, a serving provides 10% of the total carbohydrate that a "reference" person (a person who should be eating 2,000 calories a day) needs for the day. If the DV for fat on the label is 20%, then the product contains 20% of the fat that that same "reference" person needs for the day. Of course, you need to keep in mind that a child or a sedentary woman will most likely need less than 2,000 calories per day and an active teen or man may need more.

Vitamins & Minerals

These are the vitamins and minerals that appear on the label:

- Vitamin A
- Vitamin C
- Calcium
- Iron

The amounts of these vitamins and minerals are listed as a *percent* of a reference person's daily needs.

Nutrient Content Claims

Many times food manufacturers put nutrient content claims on the package. These terms are used to market the food more effectively and to set products apart from the competition. Criteria have been established by the Food and Drug Administration (FDA) for certain words, such as light and low-fat and the food must meet the criteria if these words are on the label. The FDA is trying to make it easier for consumers to understand nutrition information by making sure that products are labeled consistently. Table 7.3 features some terms and their FDA-approved definitions.

Table 7.3 FDA Guidelines for Nutrient Content Claims

Lean and extra lean	These terms are used to describe the fat content of meat, poultry, seafood, and game meats. **Lean:** less than 10 g fat, 4.5 g or less saturated fat, and less than 95 mg cholesterol per serving and per 100 g **Extra lean:** less than 5 g fat, less than 2 g saturated fat, and less than 95 mg cholesterol per serving and per 100 g
High	This term (e.g., "high fiber" or "high in calcium") can be used if the food contains 20% or more of the Daily Value for a particular nutrient per single serving.
Good source	One serving of a food labeled with this term (e.g., "good source of fiber" or "good source of calcium") must contain 10–19% of the Daily Value for a particular nutrient.
Reduced	A product labeled with this term has been nutritionally altered and contains at least 25% less of a nutrient or of calories than the regular (or "reference") product (e.g., "reduced fat" or "reduced calories").
Less or fewer	A food carrying this term on its label contains 25% less of a nutrient or of calories than a similar or reference food. Reference foods for "less" and, in the case of calories, "fewer," may use dissimilar products within a "product category." For example, pretzels may be labeled as containing "25% less fat," and this may indicate that they have 25% less fat than potato chips, not 25% less fat than other pretzels. The "product category" in this example is snack foods.

Table 7.3 FDA Guidelines for Nutrient Content Claims *(Continued)*

Light	To be labeled with this term, a product must be: 1. A nutritionally altered food containing one-third fewer calories or half the fat of the reference food. If the food derives 50% or more of its calories from fat, the reduction must be 50% of the fat calories or grams, not the total calories (e.g., "light" cream cheese has half the fat of regular cream cheese). 2. A food with the sodium content reduced by 50% (e.g., light soy sauce has half the sodium of regular soy sauce).
More	A serving of food with this word on its label, whether altered or not, contains a nutrient that is at least 10% of the Daily Value more than the reference food. The 10% or more of the Daily Value also applies to "fortified," "enriched," "added," "extra," and "plus" claims, but in those cases, the food must be altered by the manufacturer or packager.
Healthy	A "healthy" food must be low in fat and saturated fat and contain limited amounts of cholesterol and sodium. In addition, if it's a single-item food, it must provide at least 10% of one or more of vitamins A or C, iron, calcium, protein, or fiber. If the food item is a meal-type product, such as a frozen entree or a multi-course frozen dinner, it must provide 10% of two or three of these vitamins or minerals or of protein or fiber, in addition to meeting the other criteria. The sodium content cannot exceed 360 mg per serving for individual foods and 480 mg per serving for meal-type products.

Be cautious of food labeled with the terms "light" and "reduced fat." Many such foods are available on the market today and the American population is more overweight than ever! We believe that when people see this on the label they feel they can eat more of the food. If you read the label, in many instances the calories for a "light" food are almost as high as the original product! Often it is best, and even less expensive, to buy the regular product and limit portion size. Portion size is really the key to keeping calories under control.

People are very interested in organic foods. USDA passed regulations concerning organic products in 2001. Now both consumers and producers know exactly what is meant by specific terms that are given on a food label. If a product has the "USDA Organic" seal it means that it meets the criteria for "100% organic" or "organic." The USDA seal clarifies for consumers what organic means but does not imply that foods are more safe or nutritious. Table 7.4 gives the definitions of terms used for organic products.

Table 7.4 FDA Guidelines for Organic Labeling

100 percent organic	Must contain 100% organically produced ingredients, not counting added water and salt.
Organic	Must contain at least 95% organic ingredients, not counting added water and salt. Must not contain added sulfites. May contain up to 5% non-organically produced agricultural ingredients not commercially available in organic form.
Made with organic ingredients	Must contain at least 70% organic ingredients, not counting added water and salt. Must not contain added sulfites; except wine may contain added sulfur dioxide in accordance with 7 CFR 205.605. May contain up to 30% of non-organically produced agricultural ingredients.
Product has some organic ingredients	May contain less than 70% organic ingredients, not counting added water and salt. May contain over 30% of non-organically produced agricultural ingredients.

The Ingredients

While you're catching up on your reading at the grocery store, you should also take a look at the ingredients labels of your favorite foods. Federal law requires that all ingredients that are contained in a food product be listed on the label. The ingredients are listed in order by weight, from greatest to least. For example, if sugar is the first ingredient on a label, that means that by weight there is more sugar in that product than any other ingredient. There is always new research coming out about health benefits of nutrients and the government has to decide if labels should address this research. Currently, the nutrition facts label only identifies two types of fat, polyunsaturated and saturated fat. New regulations have recently been approved to include trans-fat content on the food label. This regulation goes into effect in 2006 to allow manufacturers time to alter and redesign food products and labels.

This information is important because current research indicates that we should limit our saturated fats and trans-fats and increase consumption of monounsaturated fats and polyunsaturated fatty acids. Saturated and trans-fats are associated with increasing your body's cholesterol levels and low density lipoproteins (bad cholesterol) and correspondingly increasing the risk of heart disease. On the other hand, monounsaturated fats, such as canola oil and olive oils, have been found to be beneficial to the body and may actually reduce the risk of heart disease.

Saturated fats are naturally occurring oils found in animal sources. The fat in meat, butter, milk, and in tropical oils—45% of palm oil and 70% of both palm kernel and coconut oils—is saturated fat. Unlike saturated fats, trans-fats do not naturally occur. They are polyunsaturated fats originally in liquid form that have been chemically changed by food manufacturers into their solid form. If the term "hydrogenated" or "partially hydrogenated" appears in the ingredient list, the product contains trans-fats. Current recommendations suggest avoiding these products. Margarine and shortening are trans-fats. Some food companies are already changing recipes for products, recognizing that consumers want to consume less trans-fats.

When you are shopping and reading labels, remember that polyunsaturated fats and monounsaturated fats are better choices. Polyunsaturated fats are vegetable oils such as corn oil and soybean oil. Monounsaturated fats include olive oil, canola oil, and peanut oil. We suggest that you opt for monounsaturated fats whenever possible. You will see in our recipes that we have featured these oils whenever we can.

Start the Day with Breakfast

Breakfast is the most important meal for the day—no matter what your age. It is just what the word implies, a "break" from your nighttime "fast." Most of us have dinner and maybe a snack prior to bedtime. So when we wake up, it may have been anywhere from 8 to 12 hours since our last meal. Breakfast is the meal that really gets us going in the morning and sets us up for the day. Everyone performs better when they have eaten breakfast—even if our morning meal isn't a perfectly healthy one. The bottom-line is this—EAT BREAKFAST—no matter what it is.

We should eat about 25–33% of our calories for the day at breakfast. Certain foods are often identified as breakfast foods, such as cereal or eggs, but there really is no reason you can't eat other things for breakfast or eat eggs and cereal for lunch or dinner! We list an example of a traditional breakfast and its calories in Table 7.5. You can also see how the breakfast in the table fits the nutrient needs of your child. If your family is on the run, the breakfasts listed in Table 7.6 can be eaten as they head out the door in the morning!

Table 7.5 Traditional Breakfast

Food Item	Calories	What's Good About It?
1 cup orange juice	112	Great source of vitamin C
2 scrambled eggs	199	Excellent protein source
2 slices whole wheat toast with margarine	198	Source of dietary fiber, B vitamins, and iron
1 cup low-fat milk	103	Great source of calcium
Total calories	612	

You can see how this breakfast fits the nutrient needs of your child:

	Total Calories per Day	Percent of Total Calories Provided in Traditional Breakfast
4–8 year old child	1960	31%
9–13 year old child	2794	22%
14–18 year old female	2665	23%
14–18 year old male	3543	17%

Table 7.6 Breakfast on the Run

Food Item	Calories	What's Good About It?
Apple	80	Good source of fiber
1 large bagel (4 1/2 in.)	303	Can be grabbed on the run and eaten on the bus, good source of B vitamins and iron
1 cup low-fat strawberry yogurt	250	Great source of calcium
Total calories	632	

You can see how this breakfast fits the nutrient needs of your child:

	Total Calories per Day	Percent of Total Calories Provided in Traditional Breakfast
4–8 year old child	1960	32%
9–13 year old child	2794	23%
14–18 year old female	2665	24%
14–18 year old male	3543	18%

The calorie recommendations that we have listed in Tables 7.5 and 7.6 are averages for the corresponding age groups. If you are interested in finding out the specific calorie level recommended for your child, you should visit a nutrition professional, preferably a registered dietitian. A professional will look at food intake, activity level, and growth, and determine a calorie level that is appropriate for your child. The more active your child is, the more calories he or she needs. The reverse is also true; less active children need fewer calories.

Many kids like to eat non-breakfast foods in the morning—that's fine too. Table 7.7 does the math on less-traditional breakfast items.

Table 7.7 "Nouveau" Breakfasts

Food Item	Calories	What's Good About It?
2 slices of pizza with vegetables	576	Tastes great! There are enough calories if your child is 4–8 years old but you'll need to add something if your child is older. What about a cup of juice or milk?
Ham and cheese sandwich	399	This is another good one for on-the run kids! Add a cup of low-fat milk and a cup of OJ. If your child is older or more active, what about a granola bar too?
Beef and bean burrito	254	Good source of fiber and good for the road. Your child will definitely need more calories. Add a yogurt drink!

There are many different options for a busy family to eat breakfast. Sometimes, though, even these breakfasts don't fit into your family's schedule. If this is the case, consider signing up your children for school breakfast. Many schools offer breakfast plans. In general school breakfasts are nutritionally sound and this will eliminate some of the rushing around in the morning.

Have a Healthy Lunch

Most of the year our school-aged children are eating lunch away from home. A child should have about 25–33% of their calories for the day at lunchtime. This is a recommended range of calories. The exact number of calories your child needs at each meal depends on his or her eating habits. If a child snacks frequently he or she will not need as many calories at each meal. See Table 7.8 for the details on how these numbers can translate into food choices for your children. What is the healthiest lunch? Fortunately, there are many options available for our children.

Table 7.8 How Many Calories for Lunch?

Age	Lunch-Time Calories (25–33% of Recommended Daily Calorie Intake)
4–8 year old	490–650 calories
9–13 year old	699–925 calories
14–18 year old female	666–875 calories
14–18 year old male	886–1170 calories

School Lunch

Most schools participate in the USDA-funded School Lunch Program. In order for a school to participate, it must meet certain requirements by providing a "reimbursable meal." The reimbursable meal is a complete meal. The meal must contain 33% of the calories needed for the day. Thirty percent or fewer of its total calories can be from fat and 10% or fewer from saturated fat. In addition, the menu must allow children to meet the Dietary Reference Intakes for iron, calcium, and vitamins A and C. The meal should provide increased fiber and decreased sodium and cholesterol. Although school lunch oftentimes gets a bad rap, it is a healthy choice and provides an appropriate number of calories and good nutritional value.

In many schools, the "complete meal" is offered but a child also has the option to purchase a la carte items in addition to, or in lieu of, the complete meal. Children often eat extra calories when they choose additional a la carte foods that are usually empty-calorie items like chips, cookies, ice cream, or sweetened beverages. It is easier to discourage the purchase of these items when the kids are younger, that is, in elementary school. It gets more difficult when children enter secondary school. In secondary school, they are often given even more options. At many secondary schools, a child may choose a "complete meal" or may pick and choose whatever a la carte items he or she would like. Your child can choose healthy options such as a turkey sandwich, yogurt, fruit, and milk or he or she may choose to have just French fries, cookies, and a sweetened beverage. You should encourage your child to choose the "complete" meal. If they do so, your children will receive a healthy number of calories and good nutritional value. This type of meal will also keep your child satisfied for a longer period of time.

Bagging It

Many children prefer to bring their lunch from home. If you pack your child's lunch, you have control over what is put in the lunch box! Better yet, let your child pack the lunch but make sure the options they have to choose from when they pack it are healthy ones. It is really quite easy to pack a lunch that is both healthy and satisfying. Table 7.9 features a few examples of just how to do it.

Table 7.9 Brown Bag Lunches

Food Item	Calories	What's Good About It?
Turkey sandwich on whole wheat bread with lettuce and tomato, pretzels, low-fat granola bar, banana, low-fat milk	Approximately 785 calories	Tastes great! 4–8 year olds get 40% of daily calories. 9–13 year olds get 28%. Add a pudding snack pack. 14–18 year old females get 29%. Add a pudding snack pack. 14–18 year old males get 22%. Probably needs 1 1/2 sandwiches *and* some pudding.
Sesame seed bagel, 1 cup fruit yogurt, apple, low-fat chocolate milk	Approximately 665 calories	Just grab and go! Just the right amount for a 4–8 year old. For 9–13 year old. Add 1 oz. of pretzels and a piece of string cheese. For 14–18 year old females add 2 oz. of pretzels. For 14–18 year old male add another bagel, a yogurt, and a piece of string cheese.

Food Safety

In addition to making good food choices when you pack your child's lunch, think about food safety. We're going to address food safety in more detail in Chapter 8, but you do need to think about it if you're packing a lunch.

Here are a few simple rules to follow:

- Keep cold foods cold so that bacteria doesn't grow.
  - Use an insulated bag.
  - Put an ice pack in the bag.
- Bacteria are more likely to grow in foods high in protein and water.
  - Deli sandwiches, yogurt, cut fruit, and cheese all need to be kept cold.

- Keep hot food hot.
  - Put soups, stews, and casserole-type items in a thermal container so that they maintain their temperature.

Eat Dinner as a Family

Lifestyles today are very different than they were a few years ago. We discussed several issues about busy schedules earlier in this chapter. In this section we will discuss the importance of eating together as a family unit.

It is very important to eat together as a family unit. Even if this cannot be done nightly, try to make the time at least a few times per week. Studies have shown that quality of a child's diet decreases as the child ages. This is most likely due to the fact that as a child ages more food is eaten away from home and this food is usually higher in calories and fat and lower in calcium and fiber. So it makes sense to encourage family mealtimes. Meals are also a time for the family to bond, discuss the day's events, and model good eating practices. Research indicates that children who eat family dinners have healthier eating habits! We have found that weekend breakfasts are a great time to talk over the week's activities. Why not try to have one breakfast a weekend as a family unit?

At dinner you should have approximately one third of your calories for the day, depending on your eating habits throughout the day. If you have eaten a large lunch or had several snacks, dinner should be a lighter meal. It is often at the evening meal that you want to make a concerted effort to include vegetables, because kids probably have had few, if any, servings of vegetables during the day. A typical well-balanced dinner includes an entrée or main course, a side dish, a beverage, and a dessert (fruit or something sweeter).

In Chapter 8 you will find a month's worth of menus that are easy-to-prepare and nutritious. We have also included nutritional analysis for the recipes. You will see that we often feature fruit for dessert but do list some sweeter options as well. There is nothing wrong with serving a brownie a la mode on occasion, especially if your child essentially eats a balanced healthy diet with plenty of variety. However, if your child needs to round out his or her diet by eating a dessert with a little more nutrition, offer fruit or a yogurt parfait as a sweet ending to the meal.

Have Healthy Snacks Readily Available

Eating between meals is important for growing children—adults too! It is a good idea to continually feed your body throughout the day so that your metabolism runs more efficiently. Snacking can help curb your appetite so that you are not so hungry at mealtime and overeat. The key to healthy snacking is making sure good choices are convenient and easy to choose.

It is not always easy to find "good" snacks but you want to encourage your child not to fill up on junk foods because they won't be hungry for a more nutritious real meal later. If junk food is not usually available at home they will not be able to eat it there. Again as a child gets older you have less control. So encourage your children when they are young to eat healthy snacks and get them started on the right path. Even if you child is older, though, it is never too late to start.

So what is "good" versus "junk" snack food? There really is no food that is "bad." As registered dietitians we believe that all foods can fit in a healthy lifestyle. That's right! The issue is how much and how often you eat empty calorie foods. Finding the right balance is what matters. You can't completely avoid offering sweets. Your child will end up craving these foods and as a result may overeat them whenever the opportunity arises. A child may even learn to "sneak" these foods if he or she gets the idea that these are "bad" foods. You do not want a child to come away with this idea. The most important thing is for your child to recognize that all foods can be part of a healthy diet. Moderation is the key concept in making food choices. There is nothing wrong with a candy bar. But several candy bars a day is just not a nutritious choice. Table 7.10 features some healthy snack alternatives.

Table 7.10 Healthy Snack Choices

Yogurt	Fruit
Pretzels	Granola bar
Cold cereal	Veggies and dip
Milk	Peanut butter crackers
Sports bar	Chips–try the baked ones!
Smoothie	Cheese and crackers
Bagel	Popcorn

All of the snacks in Table 7.10 are good choices, but as always, keep portion size in mind when dishing out snacks. Portion size makes all the difference. If you ate a one ounce bag of potato chips (a single-serving bag) instead of three ounces of potato chips (one third of a family-size bag) three times a week for a year, you would eat almost 47,000 calories less over the course of that year. Since there are 3,500 calories in a pound, you could lose approximately 13 pounds in a year by making this simple change (assuming the rest of your diet and your activity level did not change). It really is all about *how much you eat.* Most importantly, make it easy for your family to make good choices about snacks. Remember to keep healthy snack items easily accessible—in the front of the refrigerator and the cabinets so that your children see the healthy choices first!

Make Good Choices When Eating Out or Bringing Home Prepared Foods

People eat out more now than they ever did before. According to *Restaurants and Institutions Magazine,* it is estimated that 53% of our food dollar will be spent on food eaten away from home by 2010. Eating out is no longer considered a leisure activity but rather an essential part of our lifestyle. These days, we seem to have too much to do and not enough time to do it! So we need to be realistic and plan accordingly if we are going to take care of our family's nutritional needs. As we have discussed in previous chapters, there is nothing wrong with eating out. However, if we make poor choices by eating out too often, or always eating oversized restaurant portions, chances are we are not getting much nutrition for our calories.

There are many restaurants and even fast-food establishments that offer healthy options. For example, depending on what part of the country you're from, subs, grinders, or hoagies can be healthy choices. Many parts of the country have healthy Asian or Mexican chains. We have found that as kids age they often prefer these foods to the traditional heavy burgers and fries. Choosing appropriate portion size is important at restaurants just like at home. Children's portions are great options. They are normally a more appropriate portion size and are generally reasonably priced. Encourage your child to order these as long as possible! Above all avoid super-sized portions and consider sharing large portions. Restaurants know that people want value for their dollar. As a result of this they serve oversized portions. One serving is often enough to serve two people; so why not share the entrée or take half home and have it for another meal?

Once you've chosen your restaurant carefully and learned to consume an appropriately sized meal, make sure you order carefully as well. At restaurants, read the description of the menu item. Ask questions. Many hidden calories are in fried or sautéed foods. Order sauces and dressing on the side so you and your children can control how much is used. And watch the extras! Bread or rolls are usually on the table when you are at your hungriest and can be quickly devoured by hungry children.

Tell your server you would prefer not to have bread at your table or to bring just enough for everyone to have one piece of bread.

Many families want to eat at home but don't have time to prepare the food. "Picking up" prepared foods can be another option. Grocery stores have responded to customer needs and many now have sections that look like restaurants. Healthy options are available for you, such as roasted chicken, meatballs, fish, pasta dishes, potatoes, vegetables, and salads. Restaurants also have huge take-out businesses. This is probably a more expensive option than the grocery store deli, but at least you are eating at home and have saved on the tip!

Now back to Justin. Justin may have a breakfast program at school, which could be ideal for him. Alternatively, if he takes the bus he'll probably have plenty of time to have a healthy breakfast during his ride to school. Mom or Dad can give him something as he's running out the door. What about a bagel with peanut butter and a container of milk or juice? A granola bar or toaster pastry and a yogurt drink would also work! Justin needs to be well-fueled to meet the physical and academic demands of being a busy teen. Remember, anything is better than eating nothing for breakfast! This family needs to make some changes if they want Justin to stay healthy, but with some sensible menu planning they'll be well on their way!

CHAPTER 8

Cook It!

Now That You Have a Plan ....

Developing a good menu plan is extremely important for your family's health. As we discussed in Chapter 7, it is best if you plan in advance and have all of the foods that you think you will need for a week on hand. In addition, you should know when you will be going out or picking up dinner to eat at home. No matter what or where you choose to eat, though, you should begin by thinking about food safety. This chapter begins with some helpful hints on keeping your family safe at the dining table. We also provide you with some time saving tips and some fun ideas for encouraging your family to join you in the kitchen. And we finish up the chapter and the book with lots of tasty easy-to-prepare recipes and a sample monthly menu plan that will help get you started on the path to healthy eating in your household.

Food Safety Tips

Food safety is an important issue for everyone! It's a topic that we all need to know about. Food needs to be handled properly so that you and your family do not get foodborne diseases. The danger zone for food is 40°F to 140°F. Bacteria grow best in this temperature zone. Since you want to limit bacterial growth as much as possible, you should keep food out of the danger zone as much as possible. See Figure 8.1 for more information about safe temperatures for storing and serving food.

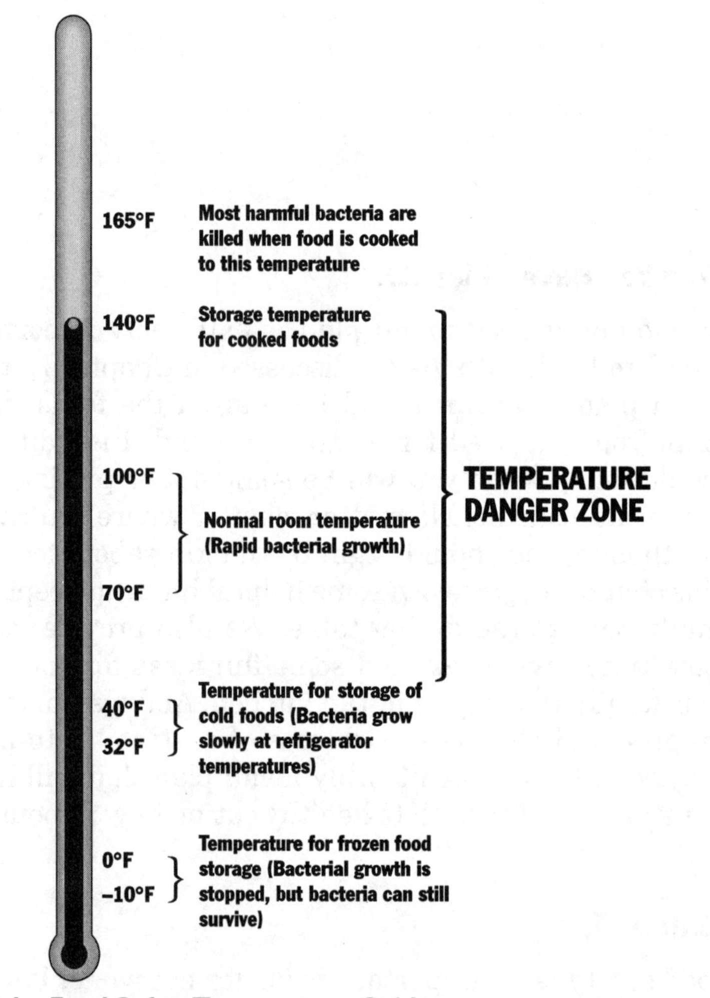

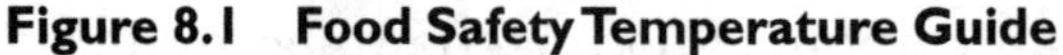
Figure 8.1 Food Safety Temperature Guide

The following are some tips for safe food handling.

Buying Food

- Make a shopping list. Put all refrigerated and frozen foods at the end of the list. Put them in your shopping cart last so they maintain a cool temperature.
- Put meat, fish, and poultry in plastic bags so that juices do not leak onto other foods in your cart.
- A "Sell-By" date indicates how long a product can be for sale.
- A "Best if Used By (or Before)" date is recommended for best flavor or quality. It is not a purchase-by or safety date.
- A "Use-By" date is the last date recommended for the use of the product while at peak quality. Make sure you will be *using* the product prior to that date.
- All meat, fish, and poultry should look and smell fresh.
- Eggs should not be cracked or broken and should be Grade A or AA.
- Make sure prepared food items are being stored under proper conditions (i.e., hot food should be hot and cold food should be cold).
- Go home right away after grocery shopping and put all items in the refrigerator or freezer immediately.

Storing Food

- The refrigerator should be at 40°F and the freezer at 0°F.
- Take food home immediately after purchasing and refrigerate it promptly.
- Freeze foods that you will not use by expiration dates.

- Put raw meat, fish, and poultry on a dish before storing so juices do not drip onto other foods and contaminate them. Put these items on lower shelves of the refrigerator.

Preparing Food

- Always wash hands in hot, soapy water for 20 seconds rubbing briskly. Rinse thoroughly and dry hands with paper towel.
- Use separate cutting boards for produce and meat. If using just one cutting board, sanitize it (with diluted bleach or in the dishwasher) after each use. Bacteria can be spread easily on cutting boards.
- Use cutting boards that are dishwasher-safe and sanitize them after each use.
- Thaw food in the refrigerator, under running water at a temperature of 70°F or less, or in the microwave if you are cooking immediately after thawing.

Cooking Food

- Cook foods to the proper temperature. See Table 8.1 for more information on safe temperatures for various foods.

Table 8.1 Safe Temperature Chart

Food Item	Temperature
Ground beef, pork, veal, lamb	160°F
Ground chicken and turkey	165°F
Beef, veal, lamb	
• Medium rare	145°F
• Medium	160°F
• Well-done	170°F
Poultry	
• Chicken and turkey, whole	180°F
• Breasts	170°F
• Thighs, wings, legs	180°F

Table 8.1 Safe Temperature Chart *(Continued)*

Food Item	Temperature
Pork	160°F
Eggs	Cook until yolk and white are firm
Egg dishes	160°F
Leftovers and casseroles	165°F

- Wash hands frequently during food preparation. Always wash hands after handling raw meats, fish, and poultry
- Never put cooked food on a dish that was holding raw meat, fish, or poultry.
- Wash knives and other utensils after they have come in contact with raw meat, fish, or poultry.

Serving and Storing Food

- Always use clean dishes and utensils.
- Never leave food on the counter to cool. Put leftovers in the refrigerator immediately. Put leftovers in containers that can be properly closed.
- Use leftovers within three to five days.
- If you freeze leftovers, put them in serving size containers so you are able to properly defrost. Use any items you freeze within two months.

Timesaving Tips

We are all very busy so we may need to take some shortcuts in order to have nutritious family meals. The following are some tips you can use to save time:

- Have frozen vegetables available—they're just as nutritious as fresh and definitely a time saver. Don't forget frozen potatoes.
- Canned fruits and vegetables are also good options and save preparation time.

- Frozen chopped onions and sliced peppers work well in recipes.
- Fresh baby carrots are a great snack and also a quick vegetable to cook—there's no peeling or cutting.
- Try doubling a recipe and freeze half—for example, make a double recipe for meatloaf and freeze one to cook later.
- Have dried spices available—if a recipe calls for fresh, substitute dried and use half of the amount.
- Slow cooker recipes are great but you need to plan ahead. Many slow cookers have a unit that separates from the cooking element so that you can put it in the refrigerator. You can put the recipe together the night before and start it in the morning.
- Do recipe preparation (peel the carrots, chop the onions and peppers, etc.) in the morning or even the night before if you can. Dinner will take less time to prepare when you get home!
- Check out your produce section—new items are being added continually. Some of the items are real time-savers. For example, pre-cut potatoes definitely save time. Salad in a bag is a great vegetable option. These convenient items can cost more, but you may be saving so much money by eating out less, you can afford to buy them now.
- Try some quick-cooking methods, such as, stir-frying, grilling, and broiling. These are not only quick but also healthy and easy to clean up!

Kids in the Kitchen

Having your child help with food preparation can be both helpful and fun! Your child may be more excited about what he or she is eating if they assist in the kitchen. The following are some ideas about what you can enlist your children do at different ages.

Three- to Six-Year-Olds

- Stir ingredients in a bowl
- Scrub and wash fruits/vegetables
- Tear lettuce
- Help gather ingredients
- Help set the table

Six- to Eight-Year-Olds

- Fill and level measuring cups and spoons
- Set the table
- Beat ingredients with a wire whisk
- Pour mixed ingredients into a prepared pan
- Use a vegetable peeler with supervision

Eight- to Ten-Year-Olds

- Open cans
- Use a microwave oven
- Prepare simple recipes with few ingredients
- Read the recipe aloud
- Gather recipe ingredients

Ten- to Twelve-Year-Olds

- Use an oven and stove top with supervision
- Use a knife with supervision
- Use a grater to shred ingredients
- Make simple baked goods
- Make a smoothie

Teens

As a teen, your child will probably be able to assist or make all of the recipes we've included in the book. Why not take advantage of your child's abilities and ask them to cook something?

Table 8.2 Your Menu Planner

Sunday	Monday	Tuesday	Wednesday	Thursday	Friday	Saturday
Roasted Chicken (use leftovers later in the week) Mashed Potatoes Gravy Green Beans Apple Walnut Crisp (recipe)	Slow Cooker Honey Glazed Pork Chops (recipe) Hash Brown Potatoes Corn Leftover Apple Crisp	Chicken and Vegetable Stir-Fry (with left-over chicken recipe) Rice JELL-O® with Fruit	Green-Chili Bake (recipe) Chopped Salad (recipe) Yogurt Parfait with Fruit*	Vegetable Soup Grilled Cheese Sandwich on Whole Wheat Bread Carrot Sticks Canned Peaches	Salmon Cakes (recipe) on Whole Grain Roll French Fries Broccoli Slaw (recipe) Fruit	Turkey Kielbasa Traditional Potato Pancakes (recipe) Sauerkraut Oatmeal Raisin Cookies
Roast Beef (use leftovers later in the week) Oven Roasted Potatoes Glazed Carrots Angel Food Cake with Strawberries	Black Bean & Vegetable Burrito (recipe) Brown Rice Fruit	Beef & Broccoli Stir-Fry (with leftover beef) (recipe) Rice Yogurt Parfait (recipe)	Pasta with Sauce Tossed Salad Warm Fruit Treat (recipe)	Slow Cooker BBQ Chicken (recipe) on a Whole Grain Roll Mixed Vegetables Chocolate-Dipped Fruit**	Penne with Tuna, Lemon, and Basil (recipe) Salad Sorbet	Chili-Cornmeal Skillet Pie (recipe) Tomato and Cucumber Slices with Vinaigrette Frozen fruit Juice Bars

Baked Ziti with Mini Meatballs (recipe) Tossed Salad Ice Cream Pie	Chicken Tenders French Fries Raw Vegetable Sticks Very Berry Shake (recipe)	Beef Stew (recipe) Bread Baked Apple	Chicken Enchiladas (recipe) Refried Beans Ice Cream	Oatmeal Pancakes with Syrup (recipe) Turkey Bacon Fruit with Pound Cake Croutons+	Fish Sticks Hash Brown Potatoes Green Beans Sliced Peaches	Frittata (recipe) Layered Nacho Salad (recipe) Pudding
Pork Chops with Sweet Potatoes and Apples (recipe) Green Beans Cool 'n Easy ® Pie with Fruit (recipe)	Pizza Tossed Salad Italian Ice	Chicken Fajitas Corn and Black Bean salad (recipe) Pudding	Scrambled Eggs Sausage Whole Wheat Toast Cantaloupe	Broccoli and Ziti Casserole (recipe) Fresh Baby Carrots Sorbet	Layered Tamale Casserole (recipe) Leftover Corn and Black Bean Salad Banana Smoothie (recipe)	Marinated Flank Steak Baked Potato Broccoli Cupcakes++

*Yogurt Parfait—Alternate layers of vanilla yogurt with fresh fruit, top with granola for a little crunch

** Chocolate Dipped Fruit—Melt semisweet chocolate morsels in the microwave and dip fresh fruit of choice – we like strawberries and bananas

+ Fruit with Pound Cake Croutons—Cut up your favorite fruit or use canned. Slice pound cake and cut into cubes. Brown the pound cake cubes under broiler and toss with your fruit.

++ Cupcakes—Try sprinkling them with powdered sugar and no frosting

Menus

In Table 8.2 we have put together four weeks of dinner menus that we hope your family will enjoy. We do not expect you to make all of the recipes in any given week, but we want to give you some ideas for quick and nutritious items that you can serve your family on a reasonable budget. The menu includes a few "breakfasts for dinner" that are very simple to make. You will see that we tried to use any leftovers for another meal later in the week. Each week there is at least one meatless meal and a really simple "kid-friendly" meal, such as grilled cheese sandwiches.

You'll find most of the recipes for the menus in the following section of the book. All of these recipes were tested and evaluated for quality in the Foods Laboratory at the University of Connecticut, Department of Nutritional Sciences. All of the nutrient analysis has been done using *Food Processor,* which is a nutrient analysis computer program often used by nutrition professionals. Each recipe has been analyzed for several nutrients. When completing nutrient analysis on the recipes, the following guidelines were used:

- If more than one ingredient is listed, the first one that appears is used for nutrient analysis. For example, if butter or margarine is an option, butter is used for analysis.
- If a range is given for a recipe (i.e., one to two cups) the first amount given (one cup) is used in the analysis.

When looking at the nutrients for a recipe, remember not to focus exclusively on that one recipe. It is better to look at intake over at least one entire day and is best to evaluate intake over several days. We hope you enjoy the meals!

Recipes

Apple Walnut Crisp

Serves 8
Active preparation time: 30 minutes
Cooking time: 40 minutes

Amount	Measure	Ingredient
1/2	Cup	All-purpose flour
3/4	Cup	Old-fashioned rolled oats
1/2	Cup	Light brown sugar, packed
1/2	Teaspoon	Salt
4	Tablespoons	Butter, softened
1/4	Cup	Walnuts, chopped
3	Pounds	Apples, McIntosh, peeled and sliced (or your choice of apple)
2	Tablespoons	Lemon juice
1	Tablespoon	Sugar

Instructions

1. Preheat oven to 375°F.
2. In a bowl mix together first four ingredients for topping. Add butter and blend until mixture looks like coarse meal. This may be done in a food processor. Stir in walnuts by hand.
3. In large bowl, toss apples, lemon juice, and sugar.
4. Spray a two-quart dish with cooking spray. Spread apple mixture into prepared pan. Crumble topping over apples.
5. Place in preheated oven for about 30 minutes or until apples are tender. Remove from oven and let sit for 10 minutes.

Nutrient analysis: 283 calories, 28% calories from fat, 12% calories from saturated fat, vitamin A 62 RE, vitamin C 2 mg, iron 2 mg, calcium 35 mg, fiber 6 g

Easy to prepare and a great source of fiber!

Baked Ziti with Mini Meatballs

Serves 12
Active preparation time: 45 minutes
Cooking time: 1 hour

Amount	Measure	Ingredient
1	Pound	Ziti pasta
1	Pound	Ricotta cheese, part skim
2	Large	Eggs
1	Cup	Mozzarella cheese, part-skim, shredded
		Marinara sauce (recipe follows)
		Mini meatballs (recipe follows)

Instructions

1. Preheat oven to 350°F.
2. Cook ziti according to package directions. Drain when cooked to desired degree of doneness.
3. Mix ricotta cheese and eggs thoroughly.
4. Place about 1/2 cup of marinara sauce in bottom of 9 × 13 inch pan.
5. Put half of the cooked ziti on top of sauce.
6. Spread ricotta cheese mixture over ziti.
7. Sprinkle meatballs throughout dish.
8. Spread about 3/4 cup of sauce, then place remainder of ziti and meatballs on top.
9. Sprinkle mozzarella cheese and about 1 cup of sauce on top.
10. Bake uncovered for about 1 hour.

Nutrient analysis: 397 calories, 33% calories from fat, 14% calories from saturated fat, vitamin A 160 RE, vitamin C 14 mg, iron 5 mg, calcium 250 mg, fiber 4 g

This is a great recipe to serve as a leftover later in the week. Just reheat in the microwave.

You will use only about half of the sauce, so you can freeze the remainder or use it for another meal.

If you don't have time to make sauce, substitute your favorite prepared jarred or canned sauce!

Marinara Sauce

Makes approximately 3 1/2 quarts
Active preparation time: 15 minutes
Cooking time: 1/2 to 2 hours

Amount	Measure	Ingredient
1	Medium	Onion, chopped
3	Cloves	Garlic, minced
2	Tablespoons	Olive oil
3	28-ounce cans	Crushed tomatoes
1	6-ounce can	Tomato paste
1/2	Cup	Red wine
1 1/2–2	Cups	Water
2	Tablespoons	Basil, dried (or 4 tablespoons, fresh)
2	Tablespoons	Parsley, dried (or 4 tablespoons, fresh)
		Salt and pepper to taste

Instructions

1. Heat olive oil in five-quart sauce pan. Add chopped onion and garlic. Sauté until wilted. Do not brown.
2. Add crushed tomatoes, tomato paste, wine, and water to make the sauce the consistency that you like.
3. Add dried basil, parsley, salt, and pepper.
4. Heat to boiling. Turn down and simmer for 1/2 hour to 2 hours.

Nutrient analysis for 1 cup: 97 calories, 18% calories from fat, 2% calories from saturated fat, vitamin A 131 RE, vitamin C 24 mg, iron 3 mg, calcium 90 mg, fiber 4 g

Mini Meatballs

Makes approximately 32 mini meatballs
Active preparation time: 15 minutes

Amount	Measure	Ingredient
1	Pound	Ground beef, 85% lean
1/4	Cup	Bread crumbs
2	Tablespoons	Parmesan cheese, grated
1	Tablespoons	Parsley, dried
		Salt and pepper to taste
1	Large	Egg

Instructions

1. Mix all ingredients together in bowl until well combined.
2. Roll approximately 1 teaspoonful of ground beef mixture into a ball. Repeat with remaining beef mixture.
3. If you are using these in the Baked Ziti recipe, you can put them in the pan raw and they will be cooked with the ziti.

Nutrient analysis per meatball: 43 calories, 56% calories from fat, 22% calories from saturated fat, vitamin A 4 RE, vitamin C 0 mg, iron 0 mg, calcium 8 mg, fiber 0 g

These meatballs are intended to go into the Baked Ziti; however, this is a great recipe for regular meatballs. It makes approximately 10 full-sized meatballs. Brown in a little olive oil before cooking in your sauce for about 45 minutes. We like to put a few raisins in the middle of the regular meatballs. They really plump up and are a great source of iron.

Banana Smoothie

Serves 1
Active preparation time: 5 minutes

Amount	Measure	Ingredient
1	Medium	Banana, ripe
1/2	Cup	Nonfat plain yogurt
1	Tablespoon	Sugar
1	Cup	Crushed Ice
1/2	Teaspoon	Lime juice

Instructions

1. Combine all ingredients in blender. Blend until smooth.
2. Serve in a large glass.

Nutrient analysis: 208 calories, 2% calories from fat, 1% calories from saturated fat, vitamin A 10 RE, vitamin C 12 mg, iron 0 mg, calcium 157 mg, fiber 3 g

A great snack or treat for dessert. Recipe can easily be doubled!

BBQ Chicken in the Slow Cooker

Serves 4
Active preparation time: 10 minutes
Cooking time: 6–8 hours on low

Amount	Measure	Ingredient
1	Cup	Ketchup
3	Tablespoons	Brown sugar
1	Tablespoon	Worcestershire sauce
1	Tablespoon	Soy sauce
1	Tablespoon	Cider vinegar
1/2	Teaspoon	Garlic powder
2		Chicken breasts, boneless, skinless (approximately 8 ounces each)

Instructions

1. Mix all ingredients except chicken breasts in slow cooker. Add chicken breasts and turn to coat.
2. Cook in slow cooker for 6–8 hours on low or 3–4 hours on high.
3. When cooked through, shred chicken with a fork.

Nutrient analysis: 238 calories, 12% calories from fat, 3% calories from saturated fat, vitamin A 67 RE, vitamin C 10 mg, iron 2 mg, calcium 35 mg, fiber 1 g

Our kids really like this served on rolls!

Beef and Broccoli Stir-Fry

Serves 4
Active preparation time: 20 minutes
Cooking time: 10 minutes

Amount	Measure	Ingredient
12	Ounces	Leftover roast beef or 12 ounces of raw flank steak
6	Tablespoons	Soy sauce
2	Tablespoons	Sherry
2	Tablespoons	Brown sugar
1	Tablespoon	Sesame oil
3	Cloves	Garlic, minced
2	Teaspoons	Ginger, chopped
1	Tablespoon	Canola oil
2	Cups	Broccoli florets
1	10-ounce package	Snow pea pods, frozen and partially thawed
6		Green onions, sliced
2	Teaspoons	Corn starch

Instructions

1. If using leftover beef, slice thin and set aside. See instructions below to prepare with flank steak.
2. Mix soy sauce, sherry, brown sugar, sesame oil, garlic, and ginger in small bowl.
3. Heat oil in wok. Cook vegetables to desired degree of doneness.
4. Stir cornstarch into marinade. Add marinade to vegetables in wok. Stir until thickens.
5. Add beef to wok and cook until heated through.

To prepare with flank steak:

1. Cut flank steak into thin slices and place in marinade. Marinade for 30 minutes.
2. Heat oil in wok. Remove steak from marinade and stir-fry until no longer pink. Reserve marinade and mix in corn starch. Place cooked beef in bowl.
3. Cook vegetables in wok to desired degree of doneness.
4. Add marinade to vegetables in wok. Stir until sauce thickens.
5. Add beef to wok and cook until heated through.

Nutrient analysis: 364 calories, 50% calories from fat, 14% calories from saturated fat, vitamin A 125 RE, vitamin C 54 mg, iron 5 mg, calcium 83 mg, fiber 4 g

This is a great use for leftovers. Good source of vitamin C and iron!

Beef Stew in the Slow Cooker

Serves 6
Active preparation time: 20 minutes
Cooking time: 10–12 hours on low

Amount	Measure	Ingredient
2	Pounds	Beef chuck, cut into 1 inch pieces
1/4	Cup	Flour
1 1/2	Teaspoon	Salt
1/2	Teaspoon	Pepper
1 1/2	Cups	Beef broth
1	Teaspoon	Worcestershire sauce
1	Clove	Garlic
1		Bay leaf
1	Teaspoon	Paprika
4	Medium	Carrots, pared and sliced
3	Medium	Potatoes, peeled and diced
2	Medium	Onions, chopped
1	Stalk	Celery, sliced

Instructions

1. Place all ingredients in slow cooker.
2. Cook on low for 10 to 12 hours or on high for 4 to 6 hours.

Nutrient analysis: 421 calories, 50% calories from fat, 19% calories from saturated fat, vitamin A 1,025 RE, vitamin C 4 mg, iron 4 mg, calcium 34 mg, fiber 3 g

Save time in the morning by cutting up the beef and vegetables (except potatoes) the night before.

Great source of vitamin A and iron!

Black Bean and Vegetable Burritos

Serves 4

Active preparation time: 15 minutes

Amount	Measure	Ingredient
4	8-inch	Flour tortillas
2	Teaspoon	Canola oil
3/4	Cup	Onion, chopped
1/2	Teaspoon	Ground cumin
1/2	Teaspoon	Chili powder
1	Cup	Chopped red bell pepper
2/3	Cup	Frozen corn kernels, thawed
1	Medium	Carrot, coarsely grated
1	15-ounce can	Black beans, rinsed, drained
1/2	Cup	Canned Mexican-style stewed tomatoes, drained
2	Teaspoon	Minced seeded jalapeno chili
2	Ounces	Monterey Jack cheese, grated (8 tablespoons)
4	Tablespoons	Sour cream
1	Teaspoon	Dried cilantro

Instructions

1. Preheat oven to 350°F.
2. Wrap tortillas in foil and warm in the oven until heated through, about 15 minutes.
3. While tortillas are warming, heat oil in large non-stick skillet. Add onion and sauté until golden brown, about 6 minutes.
4. Add cumin and chili powder; stir 20 seconds to blend.
5. Add bell pepper, corn, beans, and carrot; sauté until almost tender, about 5 minutes. Bring to simmer. Season with salt and pepper. Remove from heat.
6. Place warm tortilla on work surface.
7. Spoon filling down center of tortilla, dividing equally among all tortillas.
8. Top each with 2 tablespoons cheese. Add 1 tablespoon of sour cream and cilantro.

9. Fold sides of tortillas over filling, enclosing all the filling.
10. Turn each burrito, seam side down, onto a plate to serve.

Nutrient analysis per burrito: 366 calories, 33% calories from fat, 12% calories from saturated fat, vitamin A 605 RE, vitamin C 63 mg, iron 3 mg, calcium 262 mg, fiber 6 g

If you want to omit the sour cream, you decrease the calories to 336, fat to 28%, and saturated fat to 9%.

Good sources of vitamins A and C, iron, calcium, and fiber.

Broccoli with Ziti Casserole

Serves 6
Active preparation time: 20 minutes
Cooking time: 50 minutes

Amount	Measure	Ingredient
1/2	Pound	Ziti or other pasta shape
2	Tablespoons	Olive oil
1	Clove	Garlic, minced
1 1/2	Pounds	Broccoli, frozen and thawed
1	Pound	Ricotta cheese, part skim
2	Tablespoons	Parmesan cheese, grated
1		Egg, lightly beaten
2	Cups	Tomato sauce
1/4	Cup	Seasoned breadcrumbs

Instructions

1. Preheat oven to 350°F.
2. Cook pasta according to package directions. Drain when cooked.
3. Heat olive oil in skillet. Add garlic and sauté until softened. Add broccoli and sauté lightly.
4. In small bowl mix ricotta cheese, parmesan cheese, and egg.
5. In a 13 × 9 inch baking dish, place small amount on tomato sauce. Place half of pasta. Spread cheese mixture, then tomato sauce. Layer remaining pasta and sauce. Sprinkle top with bread crumbs.
6. Cover casserole dish and bake for 20 minutes. Uncover and bake for an additional 15 minutes until heated through.

Nutrient analysis: 373 calories, 31% calories from fat, 12% calories from saturated fat, vitamin A 193 RE, vitamin C 61 mg, iron 3 mg, calcium 271 mg, fiber 5 g

Great recipe to get the kids to eat a vegetable. Good source of vitamin C, calcium, and fiber!

Broccoli Slaw

Serves 6
Active preparation time: 10 minutes

Amount	Measure	Ingredient
1/2	12-ounce package	Broccoli coleslaw
1/2	Cup	Dry roasted sunflower seeds
1/2	Cup	Golden raisins
2	Tablespoons	Sliced almonds
		DRESSING
3	Tablespoons	Canola oil
2	Tablespoons	Cider vinegar
2	Tablespoons	Sugar
1/2	Package	Beef ramen seasoning packet
1	Package	Beef ramen noodles

Instructions

1. Mix broccoli coleslaw, sunflower seeds, raisins, and almonds in large bowl.
2. Combine ingredients for dressing. Whisk well.
3. Pour dressing on vegetable mixture and mix to combine.
4. Prior to service, crumble ramen noodles over slaw and mix to combine. Serve immediately.

Nutrient analysis: 224 calories, 52% calories from fat, 4% calories from saturated fat, vitamin A 137 RE, vitamin C 24 mg, iron 1 mg, calcium 36 mg, fiber 3 g

This is really popular with kids because of the crunch. You may think that the fat is high but the saturated fat is low. Just serve it with a lower fat entrée like grilled chicken or fish!

Chicken Enchiladas

Serves 4
Active preparation time: 25 minutes
Cooking time: 25 minutes

Amount	Measure	Ingredient
8	6 inch	Corn tortillas
8	Cups	Water
2	Cubes	Chicken bouillon
4	Pieces	Chicken breast, boneless skinless 6–8 oz (or leftover chicken)
1	Each	Bay leaf
1/2	Teaspoon	Dried oregano
2	Tablespoons	Tomato paste
1	Teaspoon	Chili powder
1	Teaspoon	Ground cumin
		Salt
		SAUCE
2	Cups	Tomato paste
		Hot pepper sauce, to taste (optional)
1/4	Teaspoon	Ground cinnamon
1	Teaspoon	Chili powder
1	Cup	Monterey Jack cheese, shredded

Instructions

1. Preheat oven to 350°F.
2. Wrap corn tortillas in foil and warm in the oven for 15 minutes.
3. Put water in large sauté pan. Add bouillon cubes and bring to a boil.
4. If using raw chicken, place chicken into broth with bay leaf and oregano. Return to boil, cover, and reduce heat to simmer. Simmer for approximately 10 minutes until chicken is done. If using leftover chicken, heat until warmed through.
5. Remove chicken breast to a bowl and shred chicken using 2 forks.
6. Add 1/2 cup of cooking liquid and tomato paste, chili powder, cumin, and salt.
7. Thoroughly mix spices throughout the chicken.

8. Combine sauce ingredients and heat through.
9. Remove tortillas from oven. Heat broiler.
10. Place chicken mixture into corn tortillas and roll up.
11. Line baking dish with enchiladas, seam side down.
12. Pour hot tomato sauce over the chicken enchiladas and top with cheese.
13. Place enchiladas under broiler for 5 minutes until cheese melts.

Nutrient analysis: 456 calories, 28% calories from fat, 13% calories from saturated fat, vitamin A 267 RE, vitamin C 20 mg, iron 4 mg, calcium 352 mg, fiber 6 g

If you want to use reduced fat cheese, you will reduce the total fat to 23% and saturated fat to 10%.

Good source of vitamin A, calcium, and fiber!

Great way to use leftover chicken.

Chicken and Veggie Stir-Fry

Serves 4
Active preparation time: 15 minutes
Cooking time: 20 minutes

Amount	Measure	Ingredient
1	Pound	Chicken breast halves, boneless and skinless, cut into 1/4-inch slices (or leftover chicken)
1/2	Cup	Bottled stir-fry sauce
1	Tablespoon	Canola oil
1 bag	12 ounces	Fresh mixed precut vegetables (broccoli, carrot, and cauliflower blend)
1	Medium	Red pepper, cut into 1/2-inch strip
1/4	Small head	Napa (Chinese) or green cabbage, cored and cut into 1-inch strips (6 cups)
1/4	Cup	Water

Instructions

1. In a small bowl, combine chicken and stir-fry sauce; set aside.
2. In nonstick 12-inch skillet or stir-fry pan, heat oil over medium-high heat until very hot but not smoking.
3. Add vegetables to skillet; cook for 5 minutes or until tender-crisp, stirring frequently.
4. Transfer vegetables to a large bowl.
5. Add pepper and cabbage to skillet; cook 5 minutes or until pepper is tender-crisp and cabbage softens. Add to vegetables in bowl.
6. If using raw chicken, place mixture into skillet and cook 4 minutes or until chicken is cooked, stirring frequently. If using leftover chicken, place in pan and heat through.
7. Return vegetables to skillet and add 1/4 cup water; cook approximately 1 minute to heat through.

Nutrient analysis: 256 calories, 26% calories from fat, 5% calories from saturated fat, vitamin A 741 RE, vitamin C 68 mg, iron 2 mg, calcium 70 mg, fiber 4 g

Great use of leftovers. Next time you make it, why not substitute beef for the chicken?

Excellent source of vitamin A!

Chili-Cornmeal Skillet Pie

Serves 4
Active preparation time: 20 minutes
Cooking time: 60 minutes

Amount	Measure	Ingredient
1/2	Tablespoon	Olive oil
1 1/2	Pounds	Ground beef, 85% lean
1	Medium	Onion, chopped
1	Medium	Green bell pepper, chopped
1	Tablespoon	Chili powder
1	Teaspoon	Minced garlic
1	15-ounce can	Chili beans
1	8-ounce can	Tomato sauce
		Cornmeal Mush (recipe follows)

Instructions

1. Preheat oven to 350°F degrees.
2. Heat oil in large ovenproof skillet over medium heat.
3. Add beef, onion, bell pepper, chili powder, and garlic.
4. Sauté until vegetables are tender and beef is no longer pink, breaking up beef with back of spoon, about 10 minutes.
5. Add drained beans and tomato sauce. Simmer until chili is slightly thickened and beef is cooked through, about 10 minutes.
6. Spoon Cornmeal Mush over chili, covering completely.

7. Place skillet in oven and bake until topping is golden brown and chili is bubbling at edges, about 40 minutes.
8. Let pie stand for 10 minutes.
9. Spoon onto plates and serve.

Nutrient analysis: 365 calories, 27% calories from fat, 9% calories from saturated fat, vitamin A 145 RE, vitamin C 26 mg, iron 4 mg, calcium 50 mg, fiber 9 g

Great fiber source!

Cornmeal Mush

Active preparation time: 30 minutes
Cooking time: 60 minutes

Amount	Measure	Ingredient
1	Cup	Yellow cornmeal
1	Tablespoon	Sugar
1/2	Teaspoon	Salt
1/4	Teaspoon	Pepper
1	15-ounce can	Whole kernel corn, drained, liquid reserved
2	Large	Eggs

Instruction

1. Preheat oven to 350°F degrees.
2. Combine cornmeal, sugar, salt, and pepper in heavy large saucepan.
3. Pour reserved corn liquid into large measuring cup. Add enough water to measure 2 3/4 cups.
4. Whisk liquid mixture into cornmeal. Add corn.
5. Using wooden spoon, stir over medium-high heat until mixture is thick and begins to boil, about 10 minutes.
6. Cool to lukewarm, stirring occasionally, about 15 minutes.
7. Mix in eggs, spread on top of Chili-Cornmeal Skillet Pie or place in buttered 10-inch diameter pie plate.
8. Bake cornmeal mixture until firm to touch, about 40 minutes
9. Let stand 10 minutes. Cut into wedges.

Chopped Salad

Serves 8
Active preparation time: 15 minutes

Amount	Measure	Ingredient
2	Tablespoons	Lemon juice
1 1/2	Teaspoons	Sugar
1	Clove	Garlic, minced
1/2	Teaspoon	Salt
1/4	Teaspoon	Freshly ground black pepper
1/3	Cup	Olive oil
1	Head, medium	Iceberg lettuce, chopped
1	Medium	Cucumber, diced
2	Medium	Tomatoes, diced
1	Medium	Green bell pepper, diced
1/4	Cup	Dried cilantro or parsley
1/4	Cup	Black olives, chopped

Instructions

1. Whisk together lemon juice, sugar, garlic, salt, and pepper in a large bowl. Add oil, whisking until combined.
2. Toss remaining ingredients in a large bowl.
3. Add dressing and mix thoroughly prior to serving.

Nutrient analysis: 291 calories, 29% calories from fat, 14% calories from saturated fat, vitamin A 243 RE, vitamin C 60 mg, iron 3 mg, calcium 237 mg, fiber 7 g

Good source of vitamins A and C, calcium, and fiber!

Cool 'n Easy® Pie with Fruit

Serves 8
Active preparation time: 10 minutes

Amount	Measure	Ingredient
2/3	Cup	Boiling water
1	4-ounce package	JELL-O® brand gelatin, any flavor
1	8-ounce can	Fruit cocktail in juice, drain and reserve 1/3 cup juice
		Ice cubes
1	8-ounce tub	Light whipped topping
1	9-inch	Graham cracker pie crust

Instructions

1. Stir boiling water into JELL-O® in large bowl. Continue stirring until completely dissolved. Add ice cubes to 1/3 cup juice from drained fruit. Add to gelatin, stirring until slightly thickened. Remove any ice.
2. Stir fruit cocktail into gelatin. Fold in whipped topping until thoroughly blended.
3. Spoon into crust. Refrigerate at least 4 hours until firm.

Nutrient analysis: 239 calories, 36% calories from fat, 18% calories from saturated fat, vitamin A 9 RE, vitamin C 1 mg, iron 1 mg, calcium 2 mg, fiber 0 g

Easy enough for the kids to make!

Corn and Black Bean Salad

Serves 8
Active preparation time: 15 minutes

Amount	Measure	Ingredient
3	Cups	Corn, frozen, thawed
1	15-ounce can	Black beans, drained and rinsed
1/4	Cup	Onion, chopped
1	Medium	Red bell pepper, chopped
1	Medium	Jalapeno pepper, seeded and chopped
1/3	Cup	Rice vinegar
1	Tablespoon	Dijon mustard
1	Tablespoon	Olive oil
3/4	Cup	Cilantro, chopped or about 1/3 cup dried
		Salt and pepper to taste

Instructions

1. In large bowl, combine all vegetables. Set aside.
2. In small bowl, mix vinegar, mustard, and oil with whisk. Add cilantro and salt and pepper to taste.
3. Pour dressing over vegetables and toss until well combined.

Nutrient analysis: 119 calories, 18% calories from fat, 2% calories from saturated fat, vitamin A 122 RE, vitamin C 33 mg, iron 2 mg, calcium 27 mg, fiber 5 g

Great side salad with good sources of vitamins A and C and fiber!

Family Frittata

Serves 4
Active preparation time: 20 minutes
Cooking time: 35 minutes

Amount	Measure	Ingredient
1	Teaspoon	Olive oil
		Cooking spray
1/2	Cup	Onion, chopped
1/2	Cup	Green bell pepper, chopped
1	Pound	Potatoes, sliced, leave skin on
3/4	Teaspoon	Salt
1/4	Teaspoon	Black pepper
4	Large	Eggs
2	Tablespoons	Dried parsley
4	Tablespoons	Salsa

Instructions

1. Heat oil in a ten-inch non-stick skillet coated with cooking spray over medium heat. Add onion and bell pepper, sauté for 5 minutes until vegetables are tender.
2. Arrange potatoes over onion mixture; sprinkle with salt and black pepper.
3. Cover and reduce heat to medium low. Cook for 20 minutes or until potatoes are tender.
4. Preheat broiler.
5. Combine eggs and parsley in a medium bowl. Whisk until well combined. Pour over vegetables.
6. Cook over medium heat for 10 minutes or until almost set. Cover skillet so that eggs will cook through. Remove from heat and broil until browned and set.
7. Cut into wedges and top with salsa.

Nutrient analysis: 233 calories, 25% calories from fat, 7% calories from saturated fat, vitamin A 108 RE, vitamin C 32 mg, iron 3 mg, calcium 55 mg, fiber 4 g

If you want to take even less time in preparation, microwave the potatoes for about 3 minutes and then slice. They will be precooked and will reduce the cooking time.

Honey Glazed Pork Chops in the Slow Cooker

Serves 4
Active preparation time: 10 minutes
Cooking time: 8–10 hours on low

Amount	Measure	Ingredient
3/4	Cup	Barbecue sauce
2	Tablespoons	Honey
3	Tablespoons	Soy sauce
1	Teaspoon	Mustard
1	Cup	Water
4	8-ounce	Center cut pork chops

Instructions

1. Combine first five ingredients in slow cooker.
2. Add pork chops and coat with sauce.
3. Cook for 8–10 hours on low or 4–5 hours on high.

Nutrient analysis: 220 calories, 26% calories from fat, 8% calories from saturated fat, vitamin A 41 RE, vitamin C 3 mg, iron 1 mg, calcium 11 mg, fiber 1 g

For variety, why not substitute a pork tenderloin or chicken?

Layered Nacho Salad

Serves 8
Active preparation time: 10 minutes

Amount	Measure	Ingredient
1	Medium	Avocado
2	Cups	Salsa
1	Head (medium)	Iceberg lettuce, chopped into bite size pieces
3	Ounces	Baked tortilla chips, broken
1	15-ounce can	Black beans, drained and rinsed
1/4	Cup	Onion, chopped
1	Small	Green bell pepper, chopped
3/4	Cup	Cheddar cheese, grated

Instructions

1. Peel and pit avocado. Mix in 1/3 cup of salsa and mash to desired consistency of guacamole.
2. In large bowl, layer 1/2 of the following ingredients: lettuce, chips, beans, onion, pepper, and cheese. Top with half of guacamole and 1/2 of remaining salsa. Repeat this layer.
3. Serve immediately or cover and chill for up to 2 hours.

Nutrient analysis: 172 calories, 36% calories from fat, 11% calories from saturated fat, vitamin A 119 RE, vitamin C 24 mg, iron 2 mg, calcium 121 mg, fiber 7 g

Good source of vitamins A and C. Excellent source of fiber!

Layered Tamale Casserole

Serves 8
Active preparation time: 20 minutes
Cooking time: 45 minutes

Amount	Measure	Ingredient
1/4	Cup	Water
2	15-ounce cans	Black beans, drained
3	Cups	Onions, sliced (about 2 large)
3	Cups	Zucchini, thinly sliced (about 2 medium)
2	Cloves	Garlic, minced
1 1/2	Cups	Red bell pepper, julienne-cut (about 2 medium)
1 1/2	Cups	Frozen whole-kernel corn, thawed
1/2	Teaspoon	Ground cumin
5	8-inch	Flour tortilla
1 1/4	Cups	Green taco sauce
6	Ounces	Monterey Jack cheese, shredded
		Cooking spray

Instructions

1. Place water and drained beans in a food processor; process until smooth. Set aside.
2. Place a large nonstick skillet coated with cooking spray over medium-high heat until hot.
3. Add onion, zucchini, garlic, and bell pepper; sauté 10 minutes. Add corn and cumin; cook 2 minutes. Set aside.
4. Preheat oven to 350°F. Coat a 3-quart round soufflé dish with cooking spray.
5. Place 1 tortilla in bottom of souffle dish. Spread 1/2 cup bean mixture over tortilla. Spoon 1 cup onion mixture over top. Top with 1/4 cup taco sauce. Sprinkle with 1/4 cup cheese. Repeat with remaining ingredients, ending with 1/2 cup cheese.
6. Bake for 45 minutes or until thoroughly heated.

Nutrient analysis: 291 calories, 29% calories from fat, 14% calories from saturated fat, vitamin A 243 RE, vitamin C 60 mg, iron 3 mg, calcium 237 mg, fiber 7 g

Some possible variations:

Use only 3 ounces of cheese and decrease the saturated fat to 9%.

Decrease both calories and fat by using reduced-fat cheese.

Substitute tomato salsa for the green taco sauce.

Oatmeal Pancakes

Serves 4 (3 each)
Active preparation time: 10 minutes
Cooking time: 8 minutes to cook all pancakes

Amount	Measure	Ingredient
1 1/4	Cups	All-purpose flour
1/2	Cup	Old fashioned or quick oats
1	Cup	Non-fat milk
1/2	Cup	Applesauce, unsweetened
1	Large	Egg, lightly beaten
1/2	Cup	Pancake syrup

Instructions

1. In large bowl, combine flour and oats. Mix well.
2. Add milk, applesauce, and egg to dry ingredients. Mix until moistened. Do not overmix.
3. Heat griddle over medium heat. Spray skillet with cooking spray. To ensure that griddle is hot enough, sprinkle a few drops of water on it. When the water drops dance, the griddle is ready for cooking.
4. Pour approximately 1/4 cup batter onto griddle. When top of pancake is covered with bubbles, turn to cook other side. (Only turn over once.)
5. Serve with syrup.

Nutrient analysis: 354 calories, 8% calories from fat, 2% calories from saturated fat, vitamin A 59 RE, vitamin C 1 mg, iron 3 mg, calcium 94 mg, fiber 2 g

Kids love breakfast for supper and these pancakes add some fiber to their diet.

Penne with Tuna, Basil, and Lemon

Serves 6
Active preparation time: 10 minutes
Cooking time: 12 minutes

Amount	Measure	Ingredient
1	Pound	Penne pasta
1	Teaspoon	Garlic, minced
3	Tablespoons	Lemon juice
1/2	Cup	Basil leaves or 1/4 cup dried
2	6-ounce cans	Tuna in oil (not drained)
		Salt and pepper to taste

Instructions

1. Cook penne according to package directions.
2. While pasta is cooking, combine garlic, lemon juice, sliced basil, and tuna with oil in small bowl.
3. Drain pasta. Put in large bowl and toss with tuna basil mixture. Add salt and pepper to taste.

Nutrient analysis: 438 calories, 25% calories from fat, 5% calories from saturated fat, vitamin A 104 RE, vitamin C 4 mg, iron 3 mg, calcium 25 mg, fiber 3 g

Simple to prepare! Tuna is a great source of omega-3 fatty acids!

Pork Chops with Sweet Potatoes and Apples

Serves 4
Active preparation time: 10–15 minutes
Cooking time: 25 minutes

Amount	Measure	Ingredient
1	Tablespoon	Canola oil
4	8-ounce	Center cut pork chops
2	Medium	Sweet potatoes (~8 ounces each) peeled and thinly sliced
1	Medium	Onion, thinly sliced
1	Medium	Apple, cored and sliced
1/2	Teaspoon	Cinnamon
1/2	Cube	Chicken bouillon
1	Cup	Boiling water
		Salt and Pepper to taste

Instructions

1. Heat large skillet. Add oil. When heated, add pork chops and brown. Remove from skillet and put on plate.
2. Add potatoes and onions to skillet. Sauté until onion is golden brown.
3. Add sliced apples and cinnamon to skillet. Return pork to skillet.
4. Dissolve bouillon cube in boiling water. Pour into skillet. Bring to boil. Reduce heat, cover, and simmer about 10 minutes until pork is cooked. Season with salt and pepper.

Nutrient analysis: 263 calories, 20% calories from fat, 6% calories from saturated fat, vitamin A 1,550 RE, vitamin C 17 mg, iron 1 mg, calcium 24 mg, fiber 3 g

Great one dish meal.

Excellent source of vitamin A.

Salmon Cakes

Serves 4
Active preparation time: 10 minutes
Cooking time: 8 minutes

Amount	Measure	Ingredient
1	14-ounce can	Red or pink salmon, drained and flaked
1		Green onion, sliced
1/4	Cup	Bread crumbs
1	Large	Egg, beaten
1/4	Teaspoon	Salt
1/4	Teaspoon	Black pepper
1	Tablespoon	Mayonnaise
1	Tablespoon	Canola oil
4		Sandwich buns, whole wheat

Instructions

1. In a medium bowl, combine salmon, green onion, 2 tablespoons breadcrumbs, egg, salt, pepper, and mayonnaise. Lightly mix with fork.
2. Shape mixture into four 3-inch round patties and roll in remaining bread crumbs.
3. Heat oil in skillet. Add salmon cakes, and cook about 5 minutes per side over medium heat until golden brown.
4. Serve on whole wheat buns.

Nutrient analysis: 448 calories, 41% calories from fat, 8% calories from saturated fat, vitamin A 59 RE, vitamin C 1 mg, iron 3 mg, calcium 260 mg, fiber 5 g

Salmon is a great source of omega-3 fatty acids!

Traditional Potato Pancakes

Serves 4
Active preparation time: 45 minutes

Amount	Measure	Ingredient
2	Pounds	Potatoes
1	Medium	Onion
1	Large	Egg, beaten
		Salt and pepper to taste
		Canola oil for browning

Instructions

1. Peel the potatoes and put in cold water. This is to prevent the potatoes from turning brown while you grate them in step 2.
2. Using a grater or a food processor, coarsely grate the potatoes and onion.
3. Place the potato-onion mixture in dishtowel and squeeze to remove as much water as possible.
4. Add the egg, salt, and pepper to the potato-onion mixture.
5. Heat a griddle or nonstick pan and coat with a thin film of oil.
6. Take about 2 tablespoons of the potato mixture in the palm of your hand and flatten as best you can. Place the potato mixture on the griddle. Flatten with a large spatula, and sauté for a few minutes until golden.
7. Flip the pancake over and brown the other side.
8. Remove to paper towel to drain any excess oil.
9. Serve immediately.

You can also freeze the cooked potato pancakes and crisp them up in a 350°F oven at a later time.

Nutrient analysis: 253 calories, 30% calories from fat, 3% calories from saturated fat, vitamin A 21 RE, vitamin C 24 mg, iron 1 mg, calcium 16 mg, fiber 3 g

Very Berry Shake

Serves 2 (8 ounces per serving)
Active preparation time: 5 minutes

Amount	Measure	Ingredient
1	Cup	Strawberries, frozen and unsweetened
1	Cup	Nonfat plain yogurt
1	Tablespoon	Strawberry jam

Instructions

1. Combine all ingredients in blender. Blend until smooth.
2. Serve in 2 large glasses.

Nutrient analysis: 120 calories, 1% calories from fat, 0% calories from saturated fat, vitamin A 4 RE, vitamin C 47 mg, iron 2 mg, calcium 168 mg, fiber 2 g

Use any berries that you like. Substitute fresh ones if in season.

Great sources for vitamin C and calcium!

Warm Fruit Treat

Serves 1 (can be made for as many as you like)
Preparation time: 5 minutes
Cooking time: 1 minute

Amount	Measure	Ingredient
1/2	Cup	Mixed fresh or canned fruit (peaches, pears, apples, fruit cocktail, banana, plums)
1	Tablespoon	Brown Sugar
1/4	Teaspoon	Cinnamon

Instructions

1. Place fruit of choice in microwaveable bowl. Sprinkle with brown sugar and cinnamon.
2. Microwave for 45 to 50 seconds until fruit is warm.

Nutrient analysis with canned peaches: 97 calories, 0% calories from fat, 0% calories from saturated fat, vitamin A 30 RE, vitamin C 5 mg, iron 1 mg, calcium 22 mg, Fiber 2 g

Great snack or dessert. Use whatever fruit you have available.

Sensible Restaurant Alternatives

In all likelihood, you will eat out or get takeout one to two nights per week. In Table 8.3 we show you what a few nights out for your family might look like nutritionally. These represent some of the better choices you can make. You'll be able to make informed nutritional choices by seeing this information. Make sure to note the serving sizes!

Table 8.3 Nutrient Analysis of Sample Restaurant Meals

Taco Bell

1 bean burrito with red sauce
1 soft taco
8-ounce low-fat milk
Nutrient analysis: 703 calories, 34% calories from fat, 12% calories from saturated fat, vitamin A 694 RE, vitamin C 2 mg, Iron 4 mg, Calcium 530 mg, Fiber 16g
Comments: Good choices. Why not end the evening with a piece of fruit?

Boston Market

BBQ chicken sandwich
3/4 cup apples and cinnamon
16-ounce soda
Nutrient analysis: 995 calories, 12% calories from fat, 3% calories from saturated fat, vitamin A 100 RE, vitamin C 0 mg, Iron 2 mg, Calcium 115 mg, Fiber 6g
Comments: Good choices. Why not end the evening with a piece of fruit?

Burger King

Chicken tenders with barbeque dipping sauce
Medium fries
16-ounce soda
Nutrient analysis: 840 calories, 34% calories from fat, 8% calories from saturated fat, vitamin A 20 RE, vitamin C 5 mg, Iron 2 mg, Calcium 15 mg, Fiber 5g
Comments: Great options for fast food! You could substitute milk for the soda to increase the calcium!

APPENDIX I

Blank CDC Growth Charts—Weight-for-Stature Percentiles

The following charts are blank weight-for-stature percentiles growth charts—one for girls and one for boys. We've chosen to include these two charts as representative for a school-aged child. You can find the growth charts for younger children as well as related charts by visiting the Centers for Disease Control (CDC) website at: http://www.cdc.gov/nccdphp/dnpa/growthcharts/training/modules/index.htm

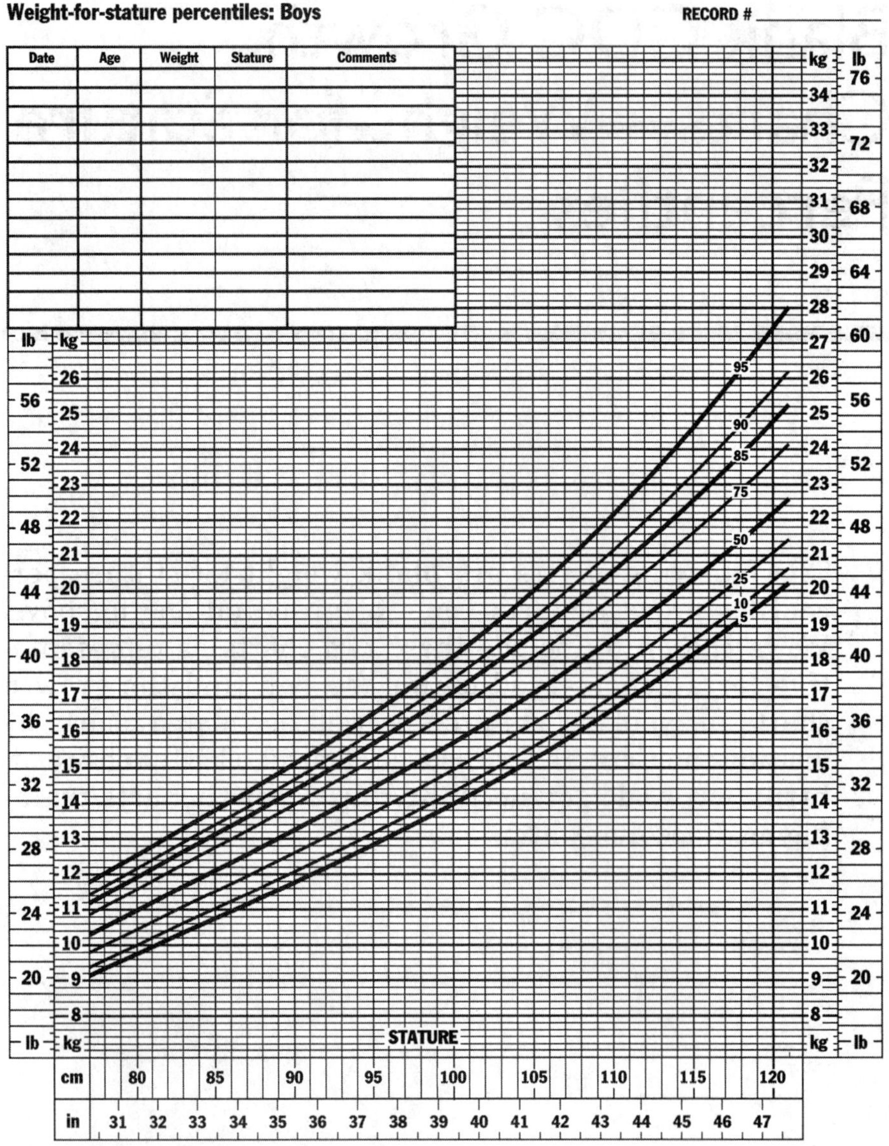

Published May 30, 2000 (modified 10/16/00).
SOURCE: Developed by the National Center of Health Statistics in collaboration with the National Center for Chronic Disease Prevention and Health Promotion (2000). http://www.cdc.gov/growthcharts

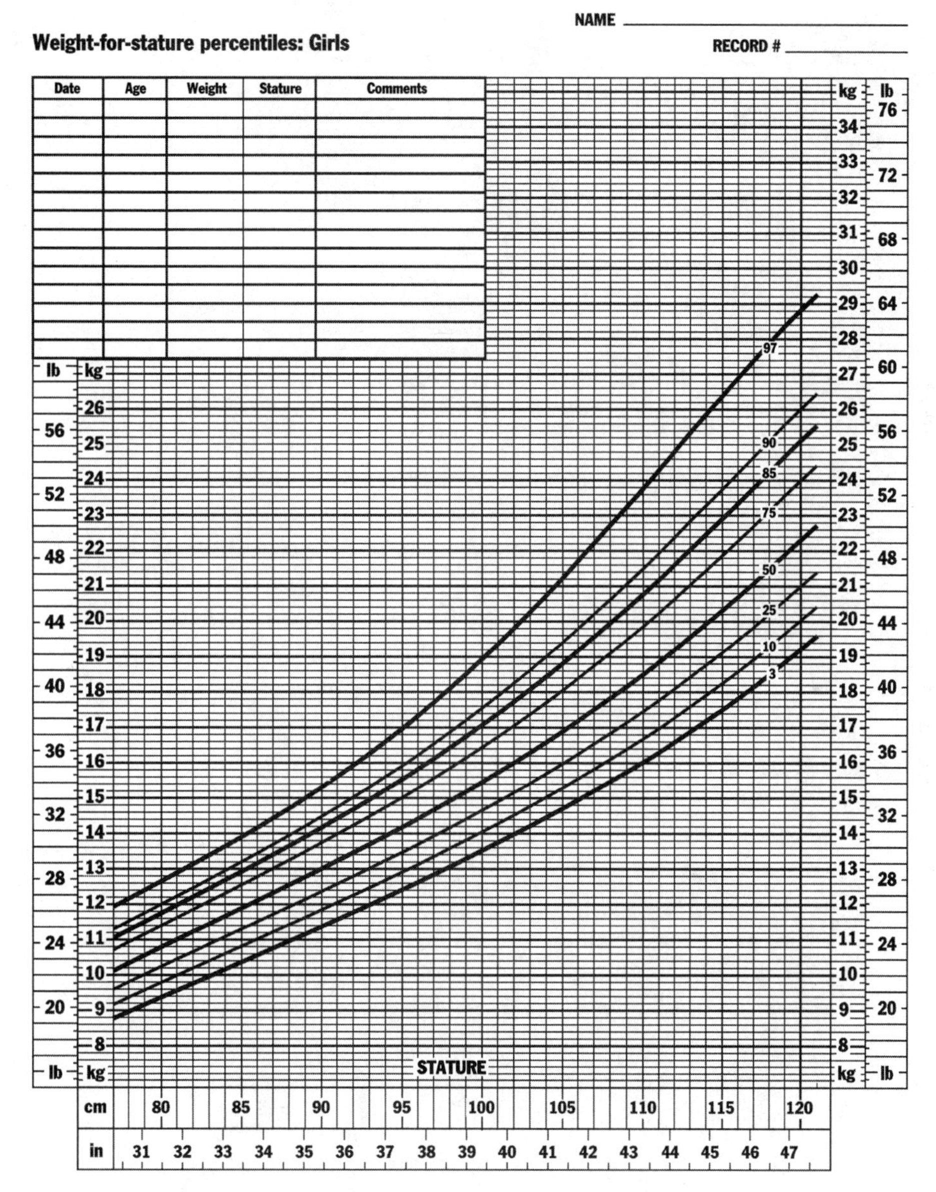

Published May 30, 2000 (modified 10/16/00).

SOURCE: Developed by the National Center of Health Statistics in collaboration with the National Center for Chronic Disease Prevention and Health Promotion (2000). http://www.cdc.gov/growthcharts

APPENDIX 2

Blank CDC Growth Charts—BMI-for-Age Percentiles

Appendix 2 includes the BMI-for-age charts for boys and girls. BMI-for-age is not used for children younger than two years of age. BMI relates weight to height using the equasion weight in kg/(height in m)^2. You can calculate BMI by dividing weight in pounds by height in inches squared and multiplying by a conversion factor of 703. round your result off to one decimal point. For example, if Sue weighs 45 pounds and 4 ounces and is 45 inches tall, her BMI-for-age is 15.7 ((45.25/45/45) $\times$ 703 = 15.7). For more information on BMI-for-age, visit the Centers for Disease Control (CDC) website at: http://www.cdc.gov/nccdphp/ dnpa/bmi/bmi-for-age.htm

CDC Growth Charts: United States

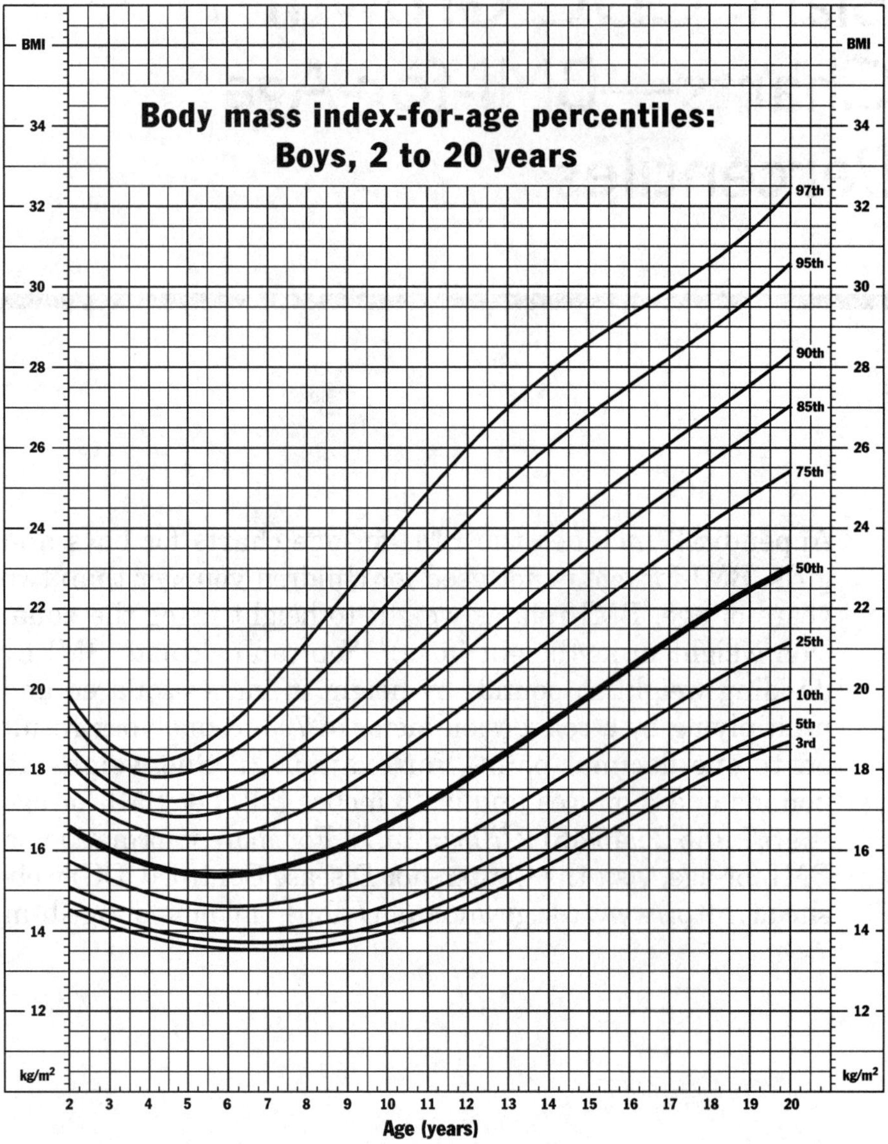

Body mass index-for-age percentiles: Boys, 2 to 20 years

BMI

34 32 30 28 26 24 22 20 18 16 14 12

kg/m²

97th 95th 90th 85th 75th 50th 25th 10th 5th 3rd

2 3 4 5 6 7 8 9 10 11 12 13 14 15 16 17 18 19 20

Age (years)

Published May 30, 2000.

SOURCE: Developed by the National Center of Health Statistics in collaboration with the National Center for Chronic Disease Prevention and Health Promotion (2000).

CDC Growth Charts: United States

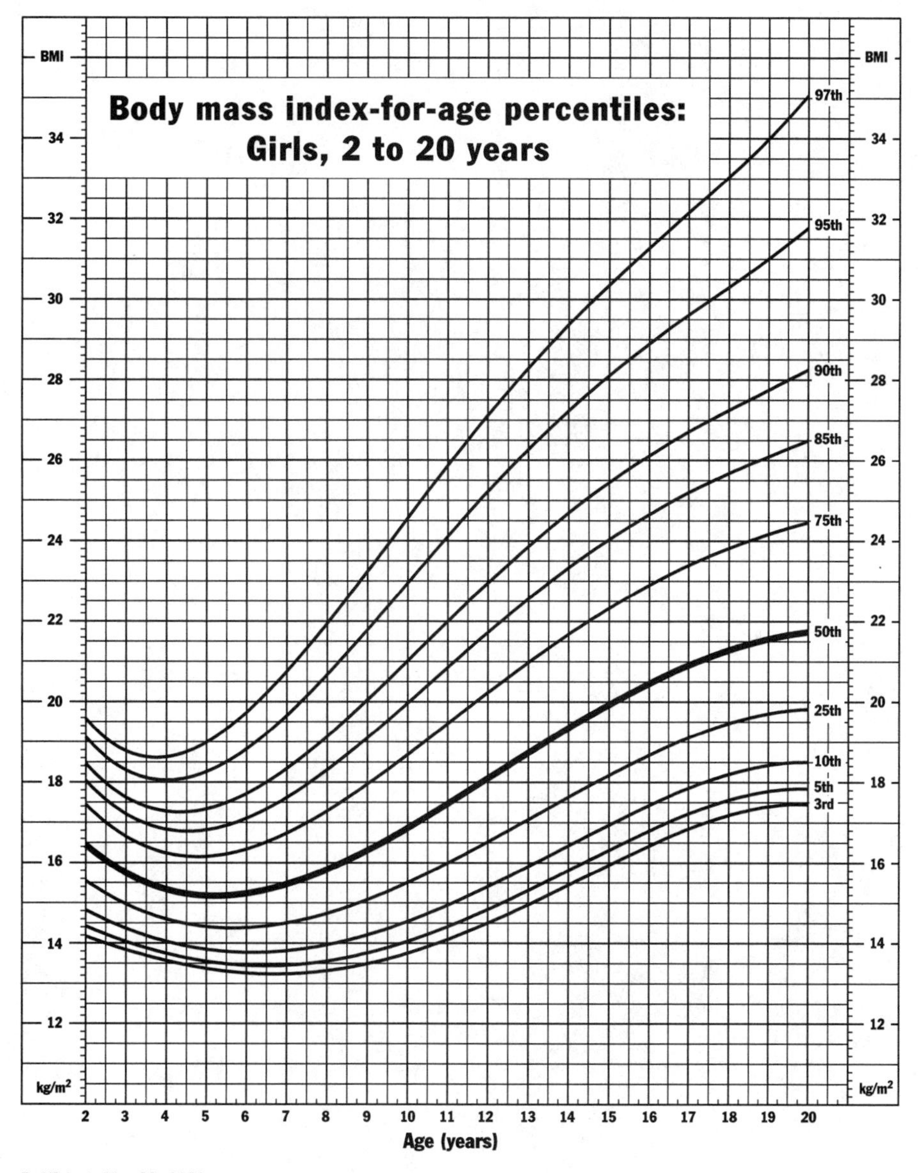

Published May 30, 2000.

SOURCE: Developed by the National Center of Health Statistics in collaboration with the National Center for Chronic Disease Prevention and Health Promotion (2000).

APPENDIX 3

Alternative Food Guide Pyramids: Latino, Asian, Mediterranean, and the Food Guide Pyramid for Young Children

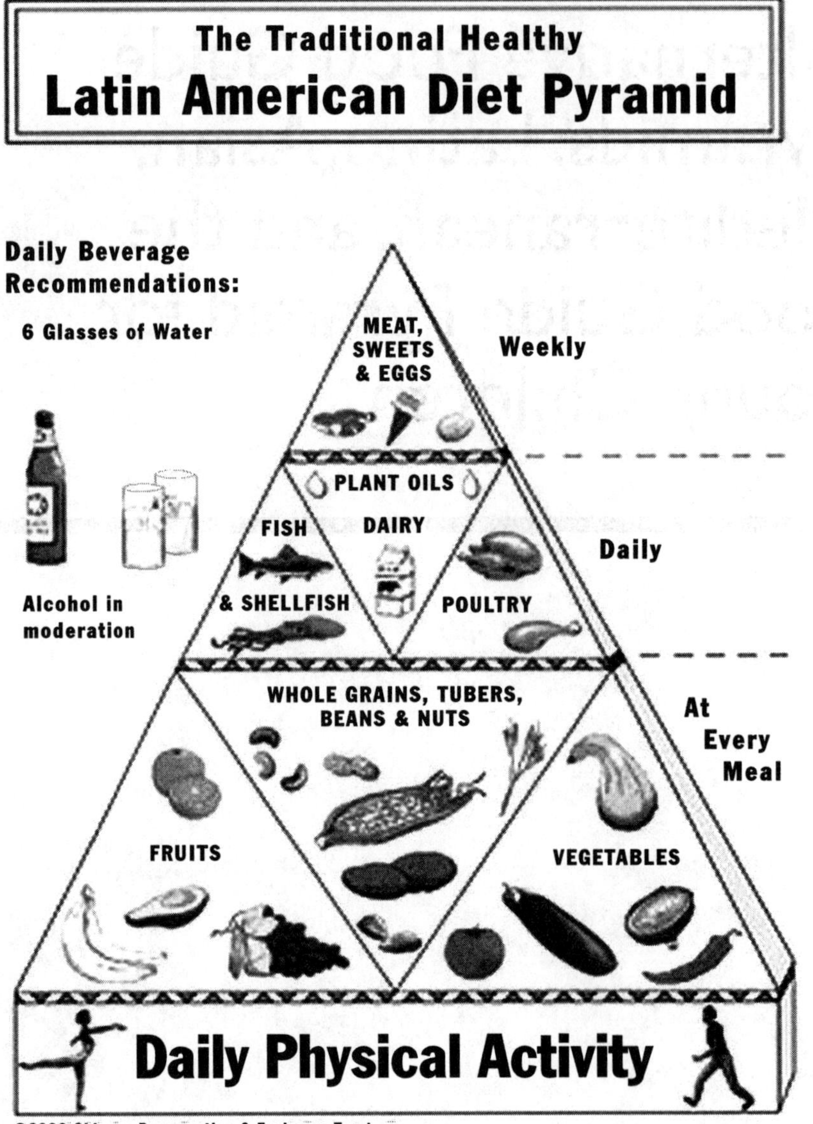
The Traditional Healthy
Latin American Diet Pyramid
Daily Beverage Recommendations:
6 Glasses of Water
Alcohol in moderation
MEAT, SWEETS & EGGS
Weekly
PLANT OILS
FISH
DAIRY
& SHELLFISH
POULTRY
Daily
WHOLE GRAINS, TUBERS, BEANS & NUTS
FRUITS
VEGETABLES
At Every Meal
Daily Physical Activity
©2000 Oldways Preservation & Exchange Trust

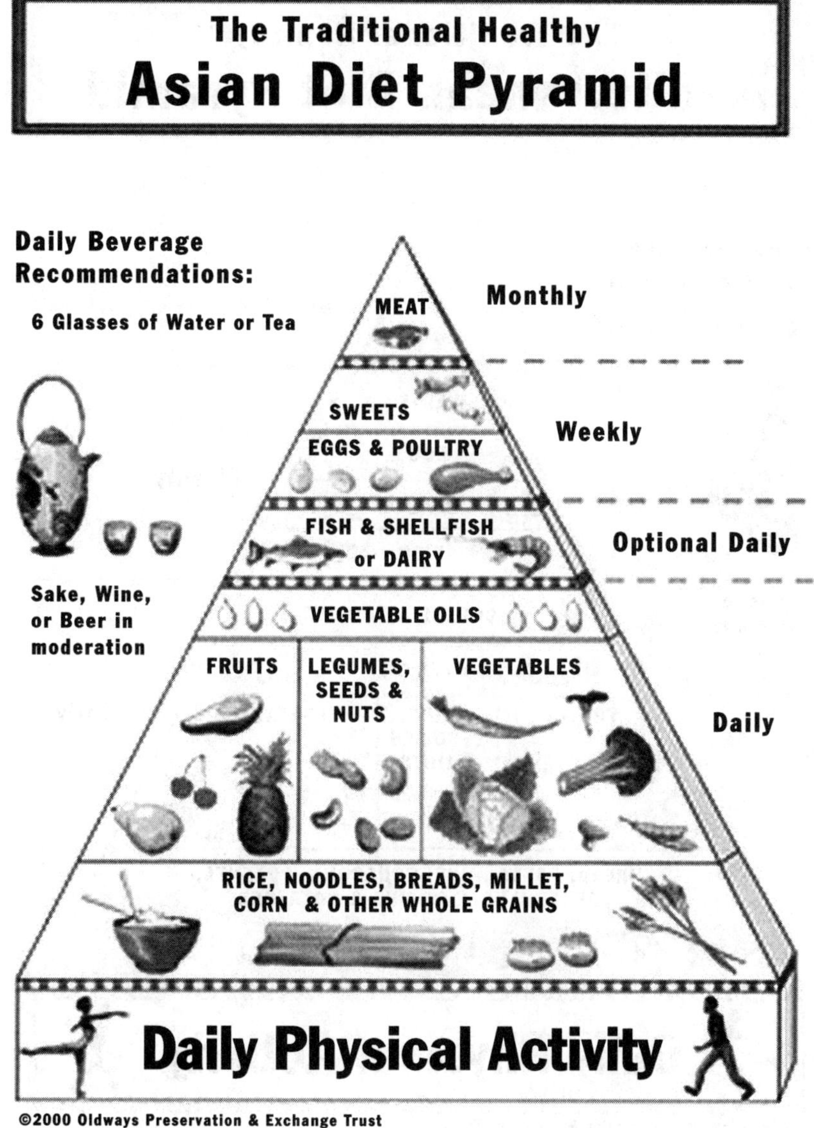
The Traditional Healthy
Asian Diet Pyramid
Daily Beverage Recommendations:
6 Glasses of Water or Tea
Sake, Wine, or Beer in moderation
MEAT
Monthly
SWEETS
EGGS & POULTRY
Weekly
FISH & SHELLFISH or DAIRY
Optional Daily
VEGETABLE OILS
FRUITS
LEGUMES, SEEDS & NUTS
VEGETABLES
Daily
RICE, NOODLES, BREADS, MILLET, CORN & OTHER WHOLE GRAINS
Daily Physical Activity

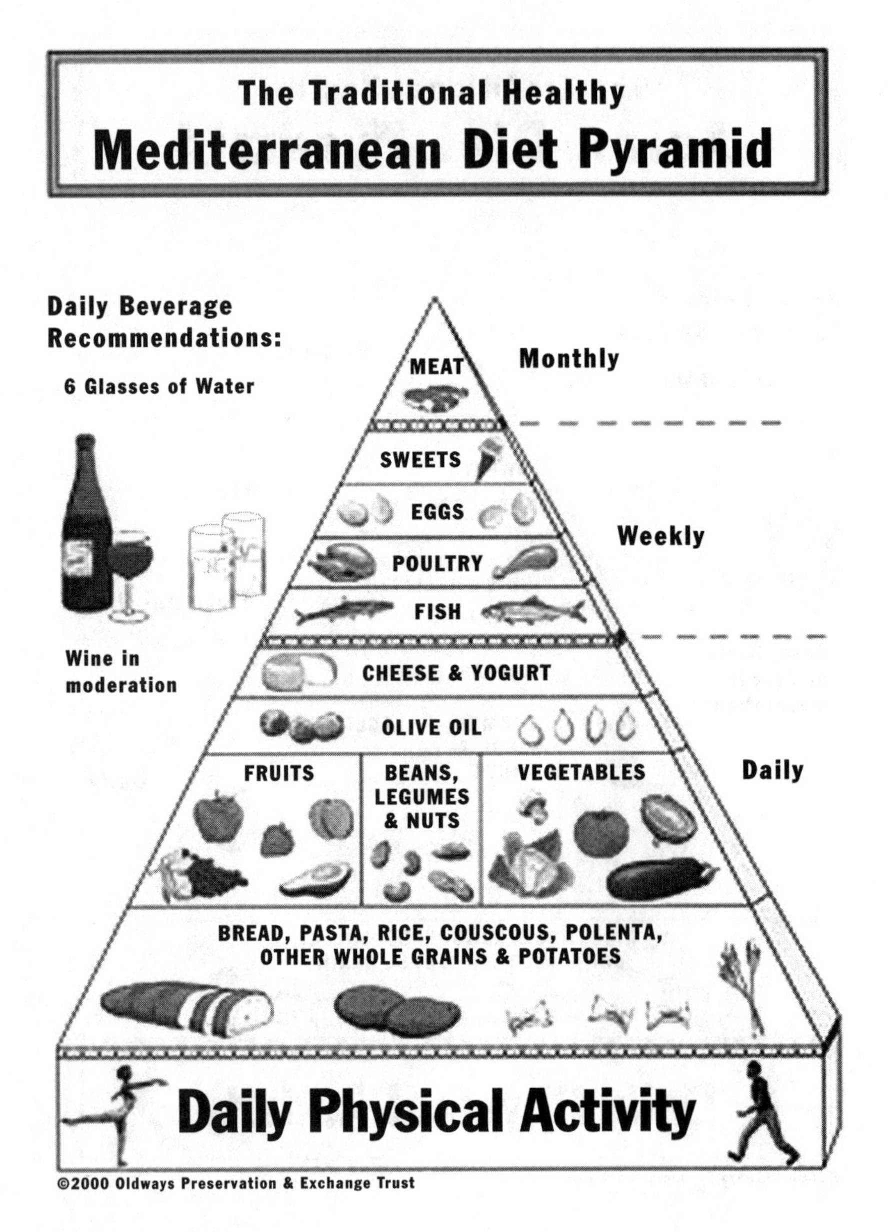
The Traditional Healthy
Mediterranean Diet Pyramid
Daily Beverage
Recommendations:
6 Glasses of Water
Wine in
moderation
MEAT
Monthly
SWEETS
EGGS
Weekly
POULTRY
FISH
CHEESE & YOGURT
OLIVE OIL
FRUITS
BEANS,
LEGUMES
& NUTS
VEGETABLES
Daily
BREAD, PASTA, RICE, COUSCOUS, POLENTA,
OTHER WHOLE GRAINS & POTATOES
Daily Physical Activity

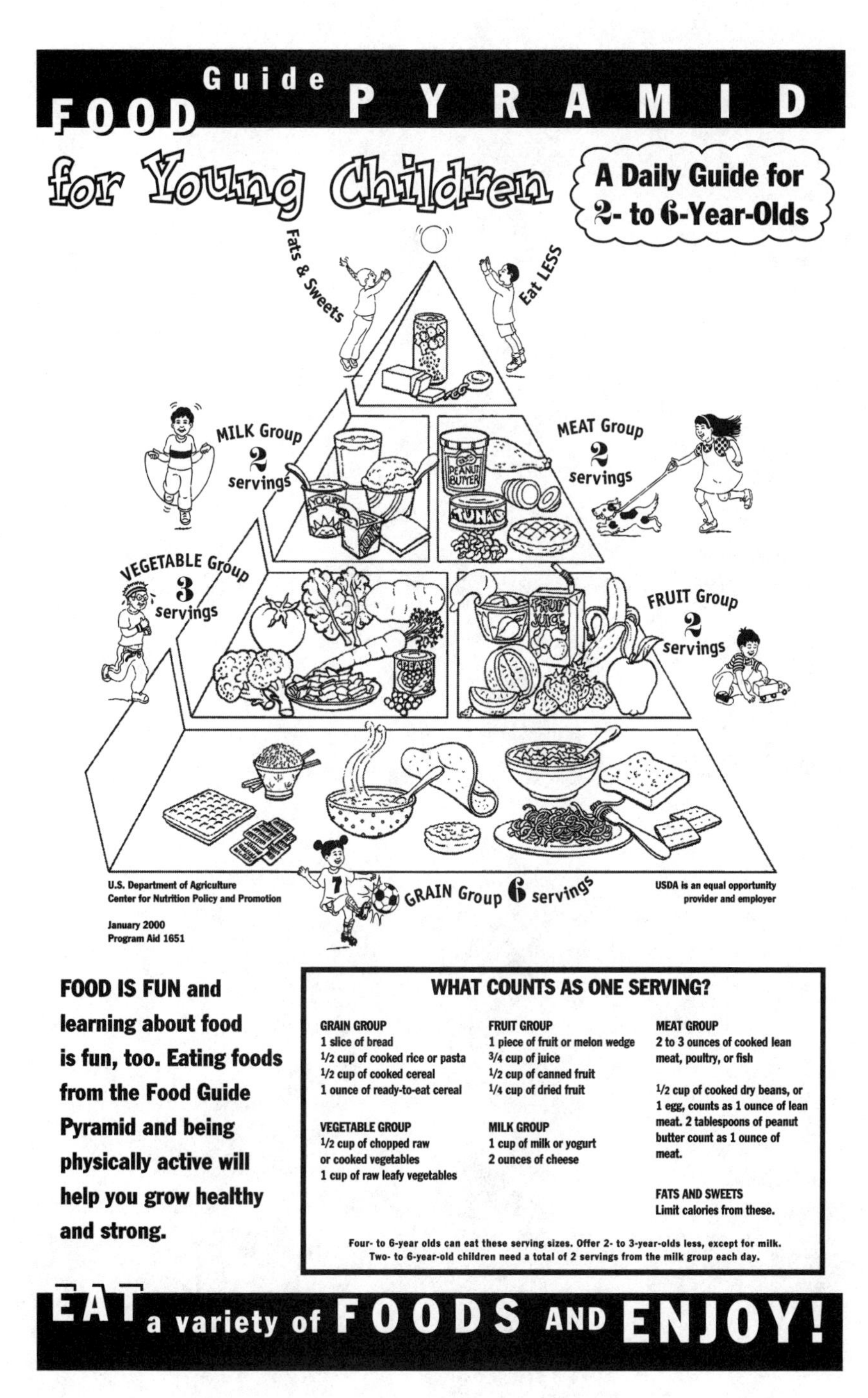
FOOD Guide PYRAMID
for Young Children
A Daily Guide for 2- to 6-Year-Olds
Fats & Sweets
Eat LESS
MILK Group
2
servings
PEANUT BUTTER
YOGURT
MEAT Group
2
servings
TUNA
VEGETABLE Group
3
servings
FRUIT Group
2
servings
FRUIT JUICE
GRAIN Group 6 servings
U.S. Department of Agriculture
Center for Nutrition Policy and Promotion
January 2000
Program Aid 1651
USDA is an equal opportunity provider and employer
FOOD IS FUN and learning about food is fun, too. Eating foods from the Food Guide Pyramid and being physically active will help you grow healthy and strong.
WHAT COUNTS AS ONE SERVING?
GRAIN GROUP
1 slice of bread
1/2 cup of cooked rice or pasta
1/2 cup of cooked cereal
1 ounce of ready-to-eat cereal
VEGETABLE GROUP
1/2 cup of chopped raw or cooked vegetables
1 cup of raw leafy vegetables
FRUIT GROUP
1 piece of fruit or melon wedge
3/4 cup of juice
1/2 cup of canned fruit
1/4 cup of dried fruit
MILK GROUP
1 cup of milk or yogurt
2 ounces of cheese
MEAT GROUP
2 to 3 ounces of cooked lean meat, poultry, or fish
1/2 cup of cooked dry beans, or 1 egg, counts as 1 ounce of lean meat. 2 tablespoons of peanut butter count as 1 ounce of meat.
FATS AND SWEETS
Limit calories from these.
Four- to 6-year olds can eat these serving sizes. Offer 2- to 3-year-olds less, except for milk.
Two- to 6-year-old children need a total of 2 servings from the milk group each day.
EAT a variety of FOODS AND ENJOY!

APPENDIX 4

Dietary Reference Intakes (DRI's): Macronutrients, Vitamins, and Minerals

The following tables are adapted from the DRI reports. We have selected key nutrients of concern (macronutrients, vitamins, and minerals) and included recommended amounts for infants through teens. For the complete tables, visit http://www.nal.usda.gov/fnic/etext/000105.html.

Dietary Reference Intakes: Macronutrients

Nutrient	Function	Life Stage Group	RDA/AI* g/d	AMDR Selected	Food Sources	Adverse Effects of Excessive Consumption
Carbohydrate—Total digestible	Role as the primary energy source for the brain; AMDR based on its role as a source of kilocalories to maintain body weight.	Infants			Starch and sugar are the major types of carbohydrates. Grains and vegetables (corn, pasta, rice, potatoes, breads) are sources of starch. Natural sugars are found in fruits and juices. Sources of added sugars are soft drinks, candy, fruit drinks, and desserts.	While no defined intake level at which potential adverse effects of total digestible carbohydrate was identified, the upper end of the adequate macronutrient distribution range (AMDR) was based on decreasing risk of chronic disease and providing adequate intake of other nutrients. It is suggested that the maximal intake of added sugars be limited to providing no more than 25 percent of energy.
		0–6 mo	60*	ND_b		
		7–12 mo	95*	ND		
		Children				
		1–3 y	**130**	45-65		
		4–8 y	**130**	45-65		
		Males				
		9–13 y	**130**	45-65		
		14–18 y	**130**	45-65		
		Females				
		9–13 y	**130**	45-65		
		14–18 y	**130**	45-65		
Total fiber	Improves laxation, reduces risk of coronary heart disease, assists in maintaining normal blood glucose levels.	Infants			Includes dietary fiber naturally present in grains (such as found in oats, wheat, or unmilled rice) and functional fiber synthesized or isolated from plants or animals and shown to be of benefit to health.	Dietary fiber can have variable compositions and therefore it is difficult to link a specific source of fiber with a particular adverse effect, especially when phytate is also present in the natural fiber source. It is concluded that as part of an overall healthy diet, a high intake of dietary fiber will not produce deleterious effects in healthy individuals. While occasional adverse gastrointestinal symptoms are observed when consuming some isolated or synthetic fibers, serious chronic adverse effects have not been observed. Due to the bulky nature of fibers, excess consumption is likely to be self-limiting. Therefore, a UL was not set for individual functional fibers.
		0–6 mo	ND			
		7–12 mo	ND			
		Children				
		1–3 y	19*			
		4–8 y	25*			
		Males				
		9–13 y	31*			
		14–18 y	38*			
		Females				
		9–13 y	26*			
		14–18 y	26*			

Total fat	Energy source and when found in foods, is a source of omega-6 and omega-3 polyunsaturated fatty acids. Its presence in the diet increases absorption of fat soluble vitamins and precursors such as vitamin A and pro-vitamin A carotenoids.	Infants			Butter, margarine, vegetable oils, whole milk, visible fat on meat and poultry products, invisible fat in fish, shellfish, some plant products such as seeds and nuts, and bakery products.	Butter, margarine, vegetable oils, whole milk, visible fat on meat and poultry products, invisible fat in fish, shellfish, some plant products such as seeds and nuts, and bakery products.
		0–6 mo	31*			
		7–12 mo	30*			
		Children				
		1–3 y		30–40		
		4–8 y		25–35		
		Males				
		9–13 y		25–35		
		14–18 y		25–35		
		Females				
		9–13 y		25–35		
		14–18 y		25–35		
Omega-6 polyunsaturated fatty acids (linoleic acid)	Essential component of structural membrane lipids, involved with cell signaling, and precursor of eicosanoids. Required for normal skin function.	Infants			Nuts, seeds, and vegetable oils such as soybean, safflower, and corn oil.	While no defined intake level at which potential adverse effects of omega-6 polyunsaturated fatty acids was identified, the upper end of the AMDR is based the lack of evidence that demonstrates long-term safety and human in vitro studies which show increased free radical formation and lipid peroxidation with higher amounts of omega-6 fatty acids. Lipid peroxidation is thought to be a component of in the development of atherosclerotic plaques.
		0–6 mo	4.4*	ND_b		
		7–12 mo	4.6*	ND		
		Children				
		1–3 y	7*	5–10		
		4–8 y	10*	5–10		
		Males				
		9–13 y	12*	5–10		
		14–18 y	16*	5–10		
		Females				
		9–13 y	10*	5–10		
		14–18 y	11*	5–10		

Dietary Reference Intakes: Macronutrients *(Continued)*

Nutrient	Function	Life Stage Group	RDA/AI* g/d	AMDR Selected	Food Sources	Adverse Effects of Excessive Consumption
Omega-3 polyunsaturated fatty acids (α-linolenic acid)	Involved with neurological development and growth. Precursor of eicosanoids.	Infants 0–6 mo 7–12 mo Children 1–3 y 4–8 y Males 9–13 y 14–18 y Females 9–13 y 14–18 y	 0.5* 0.5* 0.7* 0.9* 1.2* 1.6* 1.0* 1.1*	 ND[b] ND 0.6–1.2 0.6–1.2 0.6–1.2 0.6–1.2 0.6–1.2 0.6–1.2	Vegetable oils such as soybean, canola, and flax seed oil, fish oils, fatty fish, with smaller amounts in meats and eggs.	While no defined intake level at which potential adverse effects of *n*-3 polyunsaturated fatty acids was identified, the upper end of AMDR is based on maintaining the appropriate balance with *n*-6 fatty acids and on the lack of evidence that demonstrates long-term safety, along with human in vitro studies which show increased free-radical formation and lipid peroxidation with higher amounts of polyunsaturated fatty acids. Lipid peroxidation is thought to be a component in the development of atherosclerotic plaques.
Protein	Serves as the major structural component of all cells in the body, and functions as enzymes, in membranes, as transport carriers, and as some hormones. During digestion and absorption dietary proteins are broken down	Infants 0–6 mo 7–12 mo Children 1–3 y 4–8 y Males 9–13 y 14–18 y Females 9–13 y 14–18 y	 9.1* **13.5** **13** **19** **34** **52** **34** **46**	 ND[c] ND 5–20 10–30 10–30 10–30 10–30 10–30	Proteins from animal sources, such as meat, poultry, fish, eggs, milk, cheese, and yogurt provide all nine indispensable amino acids in adequate amounts, and for this reason are considered "complete proteins." Proteins from plants, legumes, grains, nuts, seeds, and vegetables tend to be deficient in one or more	While no defined intake level at which potential adverse effects of protein was identified, the upper end of AMDR based on complementing the AMDR for carbohydrate and fat for the various age groups. The lower end of the AMDR is set at approximately the RDA.

to amino acids, which become the building blocks of these structural and functional compounds. Nine of the amino acids must be provided in the diet; these are termed indispensable amino acids. The body can make the other amino acids needed to synthesize specific structures from other amino acids.

of the indispensable amino acids and are called 'incomplete proteins'. Vegan diets adequate in total protein content can be "complete" by combining sources of incomplete proteins which lack different indispensable amino acids.

NOTE: The table is adapted from the DRI reports, see www.nap.edu. It represents Recommended Dietary Allowances (RDAs) in **bold type,** Adequate Intakes (AIs) in ordinary type followed by an asterisk (*), and Tolerable Upper Intake Levels (ULs). RDAs and AIs may both be used as goals for individual intake. RDAs are set to meet the needs of almost all (97 to 98 percent) individuals in a group. For healthy breast-fed infants, the AI is the mean intake. The AI for other life stage and gender groups is believed to cover the needs of all individuals in the group, but lack of data prevent being able to specify with confidence the percentage of individuals covered by this intake.

UL_a = The maximum level of daily nutrient intake that is likely to pose no risk of adverse effects. Unless otherwise specified, the UL represents total intake from food, water, and supplements. Due to lack of suitable data, ULs could not be established for vitamin K, thiamin, riboflavin, vitamin B_{12}, pantothenic acid, biotin, or carotenoids. In the absence of ULs, extra caution may be warranted in consuming levels above recommended intakes.

ND_b = Not determinable due to lack of data of adverse effects in this age group and concern with regard to lack of ability to handle excess amounts. Source of intake should be from food only to prevent high levels of intake.

SOURCES: *Dietary Reference Intakes for Calcium, Phosphorous, Magnesium, Vitamin D, and Fluoride* (1997); *Dietary Reference Intakes for Thiamin, Riboflavin, Niacin, Vitamin B_6, Folate, Vitamin B_{12}, Pantothenic Acid, Biotin, and Choline* (1998); *Dietary Reference Intakes for Vitamin C, Vitamin E, Selenium, and Carotenoids* (2000); and *Dietary Reference Intakes for Vitamin A, Vitamin K, Arsenic, Boron, Chromium, Copper, Iodine, Iron, Manganese, Molybdenum, Nickel, Silicon, Vanadium, and Zinc* (2001). These reports may be accessed via www.nap.edu.

Dietary Reference Intakes: Vitamins

Nutrient	Function	Life Stage Group	RDA/AI*	UL_a	Selected Food Sources	Adverse Effects of Excessive Consumption	Special Considerations
Folate Also known as: Folic acid Folacin Pteroylpoly-glutamates	Coenzyme in the metabolism of nucleic and amino acids; prevents megaloblastic anemia.	Infants	(μg/d)	(μg/d)	Enriched cereal grains, dark leafy vegetables, enriched and whole-grain breads and bread products, fortified ready-to-eat cereals.	Masks neurological complication in people with vitamin B_{12} deficiency. No adverse effects associated with folate from food or supplements have been reported. This does not mean that there is no potential for adverse effects resulting from high intakes. Because data on the adverse effects of folate are limited, caution may be warranted. The UL for folate applies to synthetic forms obtained from supplements and/or fortified foods.	In view of evidence linking folate intake with neural tube defects in the fetus, it is recommended that all women capable of becoming pregnant consume 400 μg from supplements or fortified foods in addition to intake of food folate from a varied diet. It is assumed that women will continue consuming 400 μg from supplements or fortified food until their pregnancy is confirmed and they enter prenatal care, which ordinarily occurs after the end of the periconceptional period—the critical time for formation of the neural tube.
		0–6 mo	65*	ND_b			
		7–12 mo	80*	ND			
		Children					
		1–3 y	**150**	300			
		4–8 y	**200**	400			
		Males					
		9–13 y	**300**	600			
		14–18 y	**400**	800			
		Females					
		9–13 y	**300**	600			
		14–18 y	**400**	800			
Niacin	Coenzyme or cosubstrate in many biological reduction and oxidation reactions—	Infants	(mg/d)	(mg/d)	Meat, fish, poultry, enriched and whole-grain breads and bread products,	There is no evidence of adverse effects from the consumption of naturally	Extra niacin may be required by persons treated with hemodialysis or peritoneal dialysis,
		0–6 mo	2*	ND			
		7–12 mo	4*	ND			
		Children					

	thus required for energy metabolism.	1–3 y	**6**	10	fortified ready-to-eat cereals.	occurring niacin in foods. Adverse effects from niacin containing supplements may include flushing and gastrointestinal distress. The UL for niacin applies to synthetic forms obtained from supplements, fortified foods, or a combination of the two.	or those with malabsorption syndrome.
		4–8 y	**8**	15			
		Males					
		9–13 y	**12**	20			
		14–18 y	**16**	30			
		Females					
		9–13 y	**12**	20			
		14–18 y	**14**	30			
Riboflavin Also known as: Vitamin B_2	Coenzyme in numerous redox reactions.	Infants	(mg/d)	(mg/d)	Organ meats, milk, bread products and fortified cereals.	No adverse effects associated with riboflavin consumption from food or supplements have been reported. This does not mean that there is no potential for adverse effects resulting from high intakes. Because data on the adverse effects of riboflavin are limited, caution may be warranted.	None
		0–6 mo	0.3*	ND			
		7–12 mo	0.4*	ND			
		Children					
		1–3 y	**0.5**	ND			
		4–8 y	**0.6**	ND			
		Males					
		9–13 y	**0.9**	ND			
		14–18 y	**1.3**	ND			
		Females					
		9–13 y	**0.9**	ND			
		14–18 y	**1.0**	ND			

Dietary Reference Intakes: Vitamins *(Continued)*

Nutrient	Function	Life Stage Group	RDA/AI*	UL_a	Selected Food Sources	Adverse Effects of Excessive Consumption	Special Considerations
Thiamin	Coenzyme in the metabolism of carbohydrates and branched-chain amino acids.	Infants	(mg/d)		Enriched, fortified or whole-grain products; bread and bread products, mixed foods whose main ingredient is grain, and ready-to-eat cereals.	No adverse effects associated with thiamin from food or supplements have been reported. This does not mean that there is no potential for adverse effects resulting from high intakes. Because data on the adverse effects of thiamin are limited, caution may be warranted.	Persons who may have increased needs for thiamin include those being treated with hemodialysis or peritoneal dialysis, or individuals with malabsorption syndrome.
		0–6 mo	0.2*	ND_b			
		7–12 mo	0.3*	ND			
		Children					
		1–3 y	**0.5**	ND			
		4–8 y	**0.6**	ND			
		Males					
		9–13 y	**0.9**	ND			
		14–18 y	**1.2**	ND			
		Females					
		9–13 y	**0.9**	ND			
		14–18 y	**1.0**	ND			
Vitamin A	Required for normal vision, gene expression, reproduction, embryonic development and immune function.	Infants	(μg/d)	(μg/d)	Liver, dairy products, fish, darkly colored fruits, and leafy vegetables.	Teratological effects, liver toxicity. Note: From preformed Vitamin A only.	Individuals with high alcohol intake, preexisting liver disease, hyperlipidemia or severe protein malnutrition may be distinctly susceptible to the adverse effects of excess preformed vitamin A intake. Note: Carotene supplements are advised only to serve as a provitamin A source for individuals at risk of vitamin A deficiency
		0–6 mo	400*	600			
		7–12 mo	500*	600			
		Children					
		1–3 y	**300**	600			
		4–8 y	**400**	900			
		Males					
		9–13 y	**600**	1,700			
		14–18 y	**900**	2,800			
		Females					
		9–13 y	**600**	1,700			
		14–18 y	**700**	2,800			

Vitamin B_6	Coenzyme in the metabolism of amino acids, glycogen and sphingoid bases.	Infants	(mg/d)	(mg/d)	Fortified cereals, organ meats, fortified soy-based meat substitutes.	No adverse effects associated with Vitamin B_6 from food have been reported. This does not mean that there is no potential for adverse effects resulting from high intakes. Because data on the adverse effects of Vitamin B_6 are limited, caution may be warranted. Sensory neuropathy has occurred from high intakes of supplemental forms.	None
		0–6 mo	0.1*	ND_b			
		7–12 mo	0.3*	ND			
		Children					
		1–3 y	**0.5**	30			
		4–8 y	**0.6**	40			
		Males					
		9–13 y	**1.0**	60			
		14–18 y	**1.3**	80			
		Females					
		9–13 y	**1.0**	60			
		14–18 y	**1.2**	80			
Vitamin B_{12}	Coenzyme in nucleic acid metabolism; prevents megaloblastic anemia.	Infants	(μg/d)		Fortified cereals, meat, fish, poultry.	No adverse effects have been associated with the consumption of the amounts of vitamin B_{12} normally found in foods or supplements. This does not mean that there is no potential for adverse effects resulting from high intakes. Because data on the adverse effects of vitamin B_{12} are limited, caution may be warranted.	Because 10 to 30 percent of older people may malabsorb foodbound vitamin B_{12}, it is advisable for those older than 50 years to meet their RDA mainly by consuming foods fortified with vitamin B_{12} or a supplement containing vitamin B_{12}.
		0–6 mo	0.4*	ND			
		7–12 mo	0.5*	ND			
		Children					
		1–3 y	**0.9**	ND			
		4–8 y	**1.2**	ND			
		Males					
		9–13 y	**1.8**	ND			
		14–18 y	**2.4**	ND			
		Females					
		9–13 y	**1.8**	ND			
		14–18 y	**2.4**	ND			

Dietary Reference Intakes: Vitamins *(Continued)*

Nutrient	Function	Life Stage Group	RDA/AI*	UL_a	Selected Food Sources	Adverse Effects of Excessive Consumption	Special Considerations
Vitamin C	Cofactor for reactions requiring reduced copper or iron metalloenzyme and as a protective antioxidant.	Infants	(mg/d)	(mg/d)	Citrus fruits, tomatoes, tomato juice, potatoes, brussel sprouts, cauliflower, broccoli, strawberries, cabbage and spinach.	Gastrointestinal disturbances, kidney stones, excess iron absorption.	Individuals who smoke require an additional 35 mg/d of vitamin C over that needed by non smokers. Nonsmokers regularly exposed to tobacco smoke are encouraged to ensure they meet the RDA for vitamin C.
		0–6 mo	40*	ND_b			
		7–12 mo	50*	ND			
		Children					
		1–3 y	**15**	400			
		4–8 y	**25**	650			
		Males					
		9–13 y	**45**	1,200			
		14–18 y	**75**	1,800			
		Females					
		9–13 y	**45**	1,200			
		14–18 y	**65**	1,800			
Vitamin D	Maintain serum calcium and phosphorus concentrations.	Infants	(ug/d)	(ug/d)	Fish liver oils, flesh of fatty fish, liver and fat from seals and polar bears, eggs from hens that have been fed vitamin D, fortified milk products and fortified cereals.	Elevated plasma 25 (OH) D concentration causing hypercalcemia.	Patients on glucocorticoid therapy may require additional vitamin D.
		0–6 mo	5*	25			
		7–12 mo	5*	25			
		Children					
		1–3 y	5*	50			
		4–8 y	5*	50			
		Males					
		9–13 y	5*	50			
		14–18 y	5*	50			
		Females					
		9–13 y	5*	50			
		14–18 y	5*	50			

Vitamin E	A metabolic function has not yet been identified. Vitamin E's major function appears to be as a nonspecific chain-breaking antioxidant.	Infants	(mg/d)	(mg/d)	Vegetable oils, unprocessed cereal grains, nuts, fruits, vegetables, meats.	There is no evidence of adverse effects from the consumption of vitamin E naturally occurring in foods. Adverse effects from vitamin E containing supplements may include hemorrhagic toxicity. The UL for vitamin E applies to any form of α-tocopherol obtained from supplements, fortified foods, or a combination of the two.	Patients on anticoagulant therapy should be monitored when taking vitamin E supplements.
		0–6 mo	4*	ND_b			
		7–12 mo	5*	ND			
		Children					
		1–3 y	**6**	200			
		4–8 y	**7**	300			
		Males					
		9–13 y	**11**	600			
		14–18 y	**15**	800			
		Females					
		9–13 y	**11**	600			
		14–18 y	**15**	800			

NOTE: The table is adapted from the DRI reports, see www.nap.edu. It represents Recommended Dietary Allowances (RDAs) in **bold type,** Adequate Intakes (AIs) in ordinary type followed by an asterisk (*), and Tolerable Upper Intake Levels (ULs)a. RDAs and AIs may both be used as goals for individual intake. RDAs are set to meet the needs of almost all (97 to 98 percent) individuals in a group. For healthy breast-fed infants, the AI is the mean intake. The AI for other life stage and gender groups is believed to cover the needs of all individuals in the group, but lack of data prevent being able to specify with confidence the percentage of individuals covered by this intake.

UL_a = The maximum level of daily nutrient intake that is likely to pose no risk of adverse effects. Unless otherwise specified, the UL represents total intake from food, water, and supplements. Due to lack of suitable data, ULs could not be established for vitamin K, thiamin, riboflavin, vitamin B_{12}, pantothenic acid, biotin, or carotenoids. In the absence of ULs, extra caution may be warranted in consuming levels above recommended intakes.

ND_b = Not determinable due to lack of data of adverse effects in this age group and concern with regard to lack of ability to handle excess amounts. Source of intake should be from food only to prevent high levels of intake.

SOURCES: *Dietary Reference Intakes for Calcium, Phosphorous, Magnesium, Vitamin D, and Fluoride* (1997); *Dietary Reference Intakes for Thiamin, Riboflavin, Niacin, Vitamin B_6, Folate, Vitamin B_{12}, Pantothenic Acid, Biotin, and Choline* (1998); *Dietary Reference Intakes for Vitamin C, Vitamin E, Selenium, and Carotenoids* (2000); and *Dietary Reference Intakes for Vitamin A, Vitamin K, Arsenic, Boron, Chromium, Copper, Iodine, Iron, Manganese, Molybdenum, Nickel, Silicon, Vanadium, and Zinc* (2001). These reports may be accessed via www.nap.edu.

Dietary Reference Intakes: Minerals

Nutrient	Function	Life Stage Group	RDA/AI*	UL_a	Selected Food Sources	Adverse Effects of Excessive Consumption	Special Considerations
Calcium	Essential role in blood clotting, muscle contraction, nerve transmission, and bone and tooth formation.	Infants	(mg/d)	(mg/d)	Milk, cheese, yogurt, corn tortillas, calcium-set tofu, Chinese cabbage, kale, broccoli.	Kidney stones, hypercalcemia, milk alkali syndrome, and renal insufficiency.	Amenorrheic women (exercise- or anorexia nervosa-induced) have reduced net calcium absorption. There is no consistent data to support that a high protein intake increases calcium requirement.
		0–6 mo	210*	ND_b			
		7–12 mo	270*	ND			
		Children					
		1–3 y	500*	2,500			
		4–8 y	800*	2,500			
		Males					
		9–13 y	1,300*	2,500			
		14–18 y	1,300*	2,500			
		Females					
		9–13 y	1,300*	2,500			
		14–18 y	1,300*	2,500			
Fluoride	Inhibits the initiation and progression of dental caries and stimulates new bone formation.	Infants	(mg/d)	(mg/d)	Fluoridated water, teas, marine fish, fluoridated dental products.	Enamel and skeletal fluorosis.	None
		0–6 mo	0.01*	0.7			
		7–12 mo	0.5*	0.9			
		Children					
		1–3 y	0.7*	1.3			
		4–8 y	1*	2.2			
		Males					
		9–13 y	2*	10			
		14–18 y	3*	10			
		Females					
		9–13 y	2*	10			
		14–18 y	3*	10			
Iron (mg/d)	Component of hemoglobin and numerous enzymes; prevents	Infants	(mg/d)	(mg/d)	Fruits, vegetables and fortified bread and grain products such	Gastrointestinal distress.	Non-heme iron absorption is lower for those consuming vegetarian
		0–6 mo	0.27*	40			
		7–12 mo	11	40			

	microcytic hypochromic anemia.	Children			as cereal (nonheme iron sources), meat and poultry (heme iron sources).		diets than for those eating nonvegetarian diets. Therefore, it has been suggested that the iron requirement for those consuming a vegetarian diet is approximately 2-fold greater than for those consuming a nonvegetarian diet. Recommended intake assumes 75% of iron is from heme iron sources.
		1–3 y	**7**	40			
		4–8 y	**10**	40			
		Males					
		9–13 y	**8**	40			
		14–18 y	**11**	45			
		Females					
		9–13 y	**8**	40			
		14–18 y	**15**	45			
Phosphorus	Maintenance of pH, storage and transfer of energy and nucleotide synthesis.	Infants	(mg/d)	(mg/d)	Milk, yogurt, ice cream, cheese, peas, meat, eggs, some cereals and breads.	Metastatic calcification, skeletal porosity, interference with calcium absorption.	Athletes and others with high energy expenditure frequently consume amounts from food greater than the UL without apparent effect.
		0–6 mo	100*	ND_b			
		7–12 mo	275*	ND			
		Children					
		1–3 y	**460**	3,000			
		4–8 y	**500**	3,000			
		Males					
		9–13 y	**1,250**	4,000			
		14–18 y	**1,250**	4,000			
		Females					
		9–13 y	**1,250**	4,000			
		14–18 y	**1,250**	4,000			
Zinc	Component of multiple enzymes and proteins; involved in the regulation of gene expression.	Infants	(mg/d)	(mg/d)	Fortified cereals, red meats, certain seafood.	Reduced copper status.	Zinc absorption is lower for those consuming vegetarian diets than for those eating nonvegetarian diets. Therefore, it has been suggested that the zinc requirement for those consuming a vegetarian- diet is approximately
		0–6 mo	2*	4			
		7–12 mo	3	5			
		Children					
		1–3 y	**3**	7			
		4–8 y	**5**	12			
		Males					
		9–13 y	**8**	23			
		14–18 y	**11**	34			

Dietary Reference Intakes: Minerals *(Continued)*

Nutrient	Function	Life Stage Group	RDA/AI*	UL_a	Selected Food Sources	Adverse Effects of Excessive Consumption	Special Considerations
Zinc *(Continued)*		Females					2-fold greater than for those consuming a nonvegetarian diet.
		9–13 y	**8**	23			
		14–18 y	**9**	34			

NOTE: The table is adapted from the DRI reports, see www.nap.edu. It represents Recommended Dietary Allowances (RDAs) in **bold type,** Adequate Intakes (AIs) in ordinary type followed by an asterisk (*), and Tolerable Upper Intake Levels (ULs)a. RDAs and AIs may both be used as goals for individual intake. RDAs are set to meet the needs of almost all (97 to 98 percent) individuals in a group. For healthy breast-fed infants, the AI is the mean intake. The AI for other life stage and gender groups is believed to cover the needs of all individuals in the group, but lack of data prevent being able to specify with confidence the percentage of individuals covered by this intake.

UL_a = The maximum level of daily nutrient intake that is likely to pose no risk of adverse effects. Unless otherwise specified, the UL represents total intake from food, water, and supplements. Due to lack of suitable data, ULs could not be established for vitamin K, thiamin, riboflavin, vitamin B_{12}, pantothenic acid, biotin, or carotenoids. In the absence of ULs, extra caution may be warranted in consuming levels above recommended intakes.

ND_b = Not determinable due to lack of data of adverse effects in this age group and concern with regard to lack of ability to handle excess amounts. Source of intake should be from food only to prevent high levels of intake.

SOURCES: *Dietary Reference Intakes for Calcium, Phosphorous, Magnesium, Vitamin D, and Fluoride* (1997); *Dietary Reference Intakes for Thiamin, Riboflavin, Niacin, Vitamin B_6, Folate, Vitamin B_{12}, Pantothenic Acid, Biotin, and Choline* (1998); *Dietary Reference Intakes for Vitamin C, Vitamin E, Selenium, and Carotenoids* (2000); and *Dietary Reference Intakes for Vitamin A, Vitamin K, Arsenic, Boron, Chromium, Copper, Iodine, Iron, Manganese, Molybdenum, Nickel, Silicon, Vanadium, and Zinc* (2001). These reports may be accessed via www.nap.edu.

APPENDIX 5

Resources

Books

The American Dietetic Association. (2003). *The way to eat.* New York: John Wiley & Sons.

The American Dietetic Association. (1998). *Vitamins, minerals, and dietary supplements.* New York: John Wiley & Sons.

Dietz, W., & Stern, L. (1999). *American Academy of Pediatrics guide to your child's nutrition.* New York: Villard Books.

Duyff, R.L. (2000). *Nutrition & wellness.* New York: Glencoe McGraw-Hill.

Duyff, R.L. (1998). *The American Dietetic Association's complete food and nutrition guide.* New York: John Wiley & Sons.

Hirshman, J.R., & Munter, C.H. (1997). *When women stop hating their bodies: Freeing yourself from food and weight obsession.* New York: Ballantine Books.

Jennings, D.S., & Steen, S.N. (1995). *Play hard eat right: A parent's guide to sports nutrition for children.* Minneapolis, MN: Chronimed Publishing.

Kosharek, S. (2003). *If your child is overweight: A guide for parents,* 2nd ed. New York: John Wiley & Sons.

Melina, V., & Davis, B. (2003). *Becoming vegetarian: The complete guide to adopting a healthy vegetarian diet.* New York: John Wiley & Sons.

Pipher, M. (1999). *Reviving ophelia: Saving the selves of adolescent girls.* Putnam, NY: Econo-Clad Books.

Satter, E. (1987). *How to get your kid to eat but not too much.* Boulder, CO: Bull Publishing.

Satter, E. (1983). *Child of mine.* Boulder, CO: Bull Publishing.

Satter, E. (1999). *Secrets of feeding a healthy family.* Madison, WI: Kelcy Press.

Shanley, E.L., & Thompson, C.A. (2001). *Fueling the teen machine.* Boulder, CO: Bull Publishing.

Shield, J., & Mullen, M.C. (2002). *ADA guide to healthy eating for kids: How your children can eat smart from 5–12.* New York: John Wiley & Sons.

Stacy, L., & Mizumoto, D. (1999). *Breastfeeding: Natures best for you and your baby.* New York: John Wiley & Sons.

Tamborlane, W.V. (1997). *The Yale guide to children's nutrition.* New Haven, CT: Yale University Press.

United States Department of Agriculture and United States Department of Health and Human Services. (1996). *Food guide pyramid: A guide to daily food choices.* Home and Garden Bulletin No. 252.

United States Department of Agriculture and United States Department of Health and Human Services. (2000). *Nutrition and your health: Dietary guidelines for Americans,* 5th ed. Home and Garden Bulletin No. 232.

Websites

American Dietetic Association. http://www.eatright.org

American Academy of Pediatrics. http://www.aap.org/

Centers for Disease Control and Prevention Growth Charts. http://www.cdc.gov/growthcharts/

Centers for Disease Control and Prevention Growth BMI-for-Age. http://www.cdc.gov/nccdphp/dnpa/bmi/bmi-for-age.htm

Centers for Disease Control and Prevention Resource Guide for Nutrition and Physical Activity Interventions to Prevent Obesity and Other Chronic Diseases. http://www.cdc.gov/nccdphp/dnpa/obesityprevention.htm

http://www.fns.usda.gov/cnd/Care/CACFP/cacfphome.htm

Fight BAC! Partnership for Food Safety Education. http://www.fightbac.org/

Food Labeling and Nutrition, US Food and Drug Administration. http://vm.cfsan.fda.gov/label.html

Food Safety.gov, Gateway to Government Food Safety Information. http://www.foodsafety.gov

National Association of Anorexia Nervosa and Associated Disorders. http://www.anad.org

Nutrition Navigator: A Rating Guide to Nutrition Websites. http://navigator.tufts.edu/

Vegetarianism in a Nutshell, The Vegetarian Resource Group. http://www.vrg.org/nutshell/nutshell.htm

How to Find a Registered Dietitian in Your Area

Visit the American Dietetic Association's Website at www.eatright.org and type your zip code in the area "Find a Nutrition Professional."

INDEX

RECIPE INDEX

ABOUT THE AUTHORS

COLLEEN THOMPSON, MS, RD and ELLEN SHANLEY, MBA, RD, CD-N are registered dietitians with the American Dietetic Association and faculty members in the Department of Nutritional Sciences at the University of Connecticut. They teach several undergraduate courses in nutrition and food systems management. In addition, they have co-authored *Fueling the Teen Machine*, *Connecticut Cooks for Kids*, and numerous nutrition education articles and abstracts for a variety of professional nutrition publications including the *Journal of the American Dietetic Association*, *Journal of School Nutrition*, and the *Journal of Nutrition Education & Behavior*.

Colleen lives in Wallingford, CT, with her husband and three boys, ages 5–12.

Ellen lives in Glastonbury, CT, with her husband and two teenage children.